# 2020
# Visions

# 2020

# Visions:

## For Families, Friends, the Hopeful and the Helpful

## A book by Alan Sasala

AAS Industrial Management, Cuyahoga Community College
BA Management Systems track, Malone College
Professional Associations:
Certified State of Ohio teacher
Society of Automotive Engineers (SAE)
Certified electronics technician

Paperback ISBN: 979-8-218-26868-8
Library of Congress Number: 2023915737

First paperback edition November 2023.

Edited by Jim Scotti
Illustrations by Carl Stadtler

Reprinted by permission.

# About the Book's Cover

Frequent book readers know to never judge a book by its cover. I am hopeful that also applies to this book.

The cover's design isn't any mysterious fortune telling. The various symbols portray historical art forms from humans from both ancient and modern times. Philosophers, writers, and artists described through these art forms the symbols and thoughts from their time. They expressed themselves through art or even stories, much like Homer wrote his *Iliad* and *The Odyssey* during the Classical Greek period. **Greece after all was the cradle of democracy**.

Each of the cover's symbols are described below, beginning from the center outward.

- The grandfather clock and its hands remind us to respect time, both how wisdom springs from it and the cycle of life, birth, growth, death, and hopefully rebirth. The longer minute hand has a caduceus symbol on its opposite end. The caduceus is the staff carried by Hermes and by Iris in Greek mythology. Hermes was the herald, the wing-soled messenger and guardian of the twelve Olympians of the Greek Gods. The caduceus here acts as a counterweight on the minute hand, a reminder to keep a balanced diet to nurture our mental and physical heath. The shorter hour hand is marked with the letter *N*. The *N* represents the north needle of the mariner's magnetic compass. Its purpose is to orient people toward their destination or their way back home. The positioning of the clock's hands in the eleventh hour is to remind us that it is never too late to change a career or life path to contribute to social growth and the embodiment of wholeness. The point is to *never give up*, no matter what time it is to make those changes.

- The triangles represent life's journey and encourage you to better understand your soul and your place on earth. Triangles pointing upward represent the way to growth, prosperity, or heaven. Downward-pointing triangles represent the way to weakness, damnation, hell, or the underworld. By placing them over one another they form a hexagram. This symbolizes the Star of David and the Seal of Solomon. The Star of David has both religious and historical significance for Jewish people and the nation of Israel. In the middle of the overlapping triangles is a hexagon. Hexagons symbolize divine power, majesty, wisdom, love, mercy, and justice.

- The six pastel-colored people display various religious and social symbols: the Hebrew Star of David, the peace symbol, Christianity's cross, Islam's crescent and star, a combination symbol for men and women in marriage, and the upside-down letter *A* which symbolizes logic—acquired, natural, human common sense. They are all holding shepherd staffs. The staffs represent compassion for all that are suffering, guiding paths, authority, discipline, and defense. They were designed to protect lambs and sheep from wolves and other predators. If there were more places on the clock there would have been twelve symbols. The other six would have included the symbols for ecology, the yin-yang, and the religious symbols for Hinduism, Buddhism, Taoism, and Zoroastrianism. As a group they symbolize visibility and a need for mutual communication, respect, and coexistence; their common thread is loving humanity.

- The twelve Roman numerals are the ones typically found on grandfather clocks.

- The Eye of Providence, or the All-Seeing Eye of God, is also depicted on the US one-dollar bill and the Great Seal of the United States. The eye signifies that God is watching over humanity and to be frugal.

- The ouroboros is a snake or dragon eating his own tail. It signifies the cycle of life, death, rebirth, and infinity. The gold diamondback snake's coloring signifies how selfishness and greed for riches like gold and jewels can swallow you up and confuse your thought process and priorities in life.

- The musical symbols and instruments represent one of humanity's greatest art forms. Music historically has been a universal means for people to communicate and to share their joy. Music has been adapted by most of our world's cultural and religious practices.

# Table of Contents

# Acknowledgments

I would like to thank my family, friends, and many acquaintances for helping me with the completion of this book. A special thanks goes to my long-time friends Jim Scotti, my editor, and Carl Stadtler, the illustrator, for the many book meetings at our favorite bagel shop these past few years. Their support and belief that this book may be of interest to some, educational to others, and even a self-help guide kept me focused to get it done.

The book's cover was a group effort. It was suggested to use a local vocational school. I contacted the graphic arts department at the Cuyahoga Valley Career Center. Their talented students helped to complete the cover's copy work. Additional graphics work was done by Gary Pawlik of 3D Graphics.

However, without my wife, Karenann, continually pushing me these past few months to complete it, this book would still be in Scarlett O'Hara's "I'll worry about it tomorrow" stage. My wife's almost fifty-year companionship and her quoted adages account for many of my ideas for almost every chapter in this book.

# Prologue

It is not often that a writer begins a book, whether a prologue or introduction, with an apology. The apology is that this book took so long to finish. It is now 2024, and I began working on the notes and outline for it in 2017 with the plan of having it completed in early 2020. Hence using "2020 visions" as part of this book's title. There were many what I have been calling epiphanies that I mention throughout this book that inspired me in 2017 to begin it. When I started it, approaching the age of seventy, I had no idea that the responsibilities that come with having a large, loving family might affect the book's timetable for completion. In the end though, the extra time it took, through the daily trials and tribulations that affect everyone's life, strengthened this book's purpose. So I am so thankful for those recent good-life experiences bestowed upon me.

After preparing a preface and providing that peek into the book's content, you would think that would be enough of an introduction. However, after our planet was locked down due to the COVID-19 pandemic, a prologue was needed. Make no mistake, COVID-19 and those lockdowns have affected our "normal" routines, our thoughts, behaviors, plans, actions, and not so coincidentally, our buying habits. You have lived through it and are still living through it now. That is why so many are eager to put all the vaccinations, masking, lockdowns, and social distancing in our rearview mirrors and get back to our "normal" way of life, or what is scientifically called our "norms." I discuss norms more fully in a later chapter. My wife always looks on the bright side of things, even during pandemics, and sees a brighter future ahead for the world. She believes that working through adversities makes us stronger. I agree with her on both, and that is why I quote her often in this book.

When I first started compiling the four years of notes, memos, and research for this book, I was driven by the need to talk about how our world is focusing on too much self-gratification. For the strong of heart that is called vanity and greed. This book was meant to caution everyone to look more closely at their own selfish actions and to be more cautious about the decisions they make. However, this pandemic has caused one of the world's greatest disasters. In early 2020, my editor suggested that I get moving on the final chapters of the book because it seemed almost prophetic. This pandemic, what I call "pan-pneumonia" or the dropped C-bomb (instead of A-bomb) makes finishing this book seem so petty now. Who would have thought before November 2019 that planeloads of passengers from a virus-infected city could cause a global economic depression? With the advent of supercomputers there is no need for a crystal ball to guess what the outcome of a worldwide pandemic would be. My only hope is that I will not be judged too harshly as being sanctimonious, but understand that most of my comments were about people in 2019 BC (before COVID-19). However, the COVID effects now need to be fully scrutinized.

My editor and illustrator told me after reading the first few chapters of this book they consider it a self-help guide. Well, that was not my initial intent, but if it can help someone, anyone, I am all for that description. I know we will defeat this virus and any others that may uproot our normal routines. However, let us not make the same mistakes we made before 2020. Let us stop thinking about "me first," and let's all do more to recognize our social problems. In chapter 1 I tell how I believe in *observation not discrimination* and use the dictionary's definition for each (at least while the dictionary's descriptions are not all uprooted). I explain the differences between them and how we must approach all issues with an open mind, analyze the important ones, and digest as many factors as possible before deciding on them. Make decisions that will benefit all. That is what I hope and pray for. We are all God's children, and not any one of us is any better than the other, no matter how much someone or some group may think otherwise. Egos and envy are dangerous things. I believe if we all just take a little more time to research some important issues, even as little as our personal or family budgets, those issues will make our nation the best ever and lead us to bountiful improvements that other nations will want to follow. Those improvements are discussed in more detail in the last chapter, "A New Age for Reasoning."

Discussed in the preface and chapter 1 is how our American music profoundly affected my life. So much so, it was our American music that also inspired me to write this book. At the end of each chapter I give credit to a song or two that made me think about the chapter's subject matter. For this prologue it was the song "Help" by the Beatles, which was performed by the Beatles and written by John Lennon and Paul McCartney, and "Raindrops Keep Fallin' on My Head," sung by B. J. Thomas and written by Burt F. Bacharach and Hal David. In "Help" the Beatles sing that they are down, confused by too many changes, and seem to lose their independence through confusion. They know that people can help them and appreciate their help. In "Raindrops Keep Fallin' on My Head," B. J. Thomas sings about rain falling on his head but knows it is only temporary (as being stuck in a pandemic). The sun will shine again, and the sadness that came with the rain or any tragedy will pass in time, so there isn't any need to worry about it because good people will fix it. Many wise leaders have said these words, "It is easy for evil to prevail if good men (people) do nothing." Evil people or nations always go to the scare tactic or terrorizing people to make their targets fold and go into hiding or running from any confrontation. The most recent activist religious leader, Pope John Paul II, often gave these words of encouragement. [1]He said, "Be not afraid." [2]He was referencing the many times those words, "Do not be afraid" are quoted in the Bible.

I enjoy listening to these inspirational songs I reference after each chapter and appreciate the hard work the writers and performing artists put into them. I imagine their motivation for their artistry is attributed to some of their beliefs or the trials, tribulations, or hopefully jubilations they experienced and wanted to share through their songs.

# Preface

It is only fitting in these high-tech, social, and multimedia-blitz times that I tell you, "I am not a robot." I am a humanoid of the planet Earth, from which all these great wonders of life have been created. You need to know that because of all the internet hacking and AI (artificial intelligence), viruses and identity theft are occurring without any end in sight. Also know that I am beholden to the earthlings known as mother and father, and to God, for doing their part in this creation. So much for my disclaimer.

I was born in 1953 in Cleveland, Ohio, and grew up in the inner city. My upbringing was purely part of the great American middle class, and music was woven into my life's fiber. Music was always played in our home or in our car. It could be through record players, my older brother or sister's transistor radios, or my father's accordion. We listened to a variety of music and enjoyed it all. We heard my mother and father's record players. My dad's favorite music was by Al Jolson and Jerry Vale. My mom often played her old 78-speed records from country and western stars Hank Williams and Hank Snow, or the Mills Brothers and the Ink Spots jazz music.

Thanks to DJ Alan Freed, Cleveland was a big rock 'n' roll town. My brother and sister and I were all into rock 'n' roll. As a pre-teen I remember listening to the Big Bopper and doo-wop stuff, all the way to Motown. In the '60s the music ranged from the Four Seasons and the Lettermen to the Beatles and the Rolling Stones.

Music always had big impact on my life, and later as a teenager I recorded my favorite songs and played them everywhere I went. When I was a senior in high school the movie *Love Story* had just come out. My English teacher gave us an assignment about the movie and what it meant to us. At that time, I was a huge Jimi Hendrix fan and had just learned of his death. I wondered why he overdosed on drugs and thought that it could have been caused by a broken heart. For the assignment I compiled many of Jimi's lyrics and arranged them into a story I titled "Love Story," about how he met his girlfriend and how they fell into and then out of love. So, the "out of love" was the end of the assignment and the end of Jimi's life, along with Ali McGraw's character in the movie of the same name. The assignment took a long to time complete, but like most things in life, the hard work produced an A grade. Later, in college, after meeting and dating my wife, I tape recorded her favorite country and rock music artists' songs for her to listen to at anytime and anywhere.

I am telling a similar story in this book about how I see humanity in our world today, how I was raised, the importance of our families, making ends meet for ourselves and our children, and the grind of our society. The various types of music I listened to left an impression on me. Certain performing artists and song lyrics told me more about life's experiences than anything else I was exposed to. I'm sure plays, movies, or books by Shakespeare or Charles Dickens or even the Bible may have positively affected your life in some ways. The music helped shape mine. I see some things today and wonder what could possibly have led to the decisions made on important issues, and I try to scientifically reason them out. Some of the topics are funny, others a little more serious. I hope my many observations from this book will positively affect you and hopefully help sustain our great American middle class, making it fairer and freer. In each chapter I give credit to the music that inspired it. I tell a little bit about what the artists' message may mean and how my eyes have seen some related events. What else would you expect from a kid from Cleveland, the rock 'n' roll capital of the world?

I am hopeful, as my 2020 title implies, to open your eyes to the many things affecting our families and friends today. My eyes have seen many things for nearly fifty years in the twentieth century and now have seen things for over twenty years in the twenty-first century. There is a definite, almost scary dichotomy of the decisions made by people in these two centuries. As a history buff, my concerns are that the many distractions thrown at us today, almost like a blitzkrieg from all directions, may be clouding our ability to take the time to decipher each important event.

Every current event should be given the time for us to analyze the many factors in each to help us make educated decisions instead of using the "group loyalty knee-jerk" process. Hey, if some dummy posts a note to his or her thread on the internet, or tweets about packing a mall at a certain time, the next thing you know, a riot breaks out. It is like, "Let's all storm the Bastille." It is not just the riot itself that concerns me, it is the high-tech tools used to "get the message out" to their gangs that should concern people. Joining in these "knee-jerk" mob scenes appears to be fulfilling fantasies about one's own existence. This prevailing attitude today has caused me to label the twenty-first century as "the century of self-fulfilling prophecies." This label came about from my observations while working for many years in public service. Many people often describe public service as self-serving, which can and has happened. We can't afford for our elected officials to use our tax money for their own agendas instead of what is beneficial for *us*, the tax-paying voters, not *them*. This is not only my observation, but I believe you have seen these actions by many of our elected officials as well.

This book contains many of my observations. Again, I am a history buff, but I also pride myself in being scientific. Most of my observations in this book are made in a purposeful, scientific manner. Your opinions or judgments about these observations are purely your own. Perhaps you may detect a bit of sarcasm from some. *It is meant to entertain you.* I like to have fun too! My wife always says, "There's a little bit of truth in every sarcasm." Like the very popular 1970s TV police mystery series that starred Peter Faulk, I often quote my wife throughout this book, as with others who have greatly affected my life.

This book purposely makes the grave mistake of mentioning subjects that we have been told to *never* mention in public due to the potential for (heaven forbid) a debate. Mentioned here are the unmentionables of politics, religion, sex, money, and even unions. The other hair-raising subjects are love, hate, rights, parenting, drugs, education, sports, social media, journalism, entertainment, family, government, culture, race, and ethics. Let us call it an exercise in the American's First Amendment right to free speech.

I repeatedly use many phrases from my observations such as: "beholden," being "found out," "enabling," "condition response," "the scientific method," "tail wagging the dog," "paying the piper to call the tune," "Big Brother," "perception and reality," "painted into a corner" (entrapment), "the shell game" (distractions), being "bull-jived" and "politically guilted" (shamed), and "the media's cultivation of racial hate."

I hope you enjoy reading this book as much as I have enjoyed writing it. I mentioned that I enjoyed the music that inspired me to write it even more! For this chapter, my inspiration came from the song "Double Vision." It was written by Lou Gramm and Mick Jones and performed by the rock group Foreigner. The song encapsulates the essences of this book and the dichotomy of two centuries. For me, the double vision is about how the information we are receiving though our various media may be purposely creating more polarization in politics and causing all of us to be more and more dysfunctional, confused, and cross-eyed. This is purely my observation over the past few years. I could give an opinion on why it is happening, but I would rather have the conduits of information we receive today, like the television and internet gurus, just correct their abuse. Should the media continue to obfuscate information, my only hope is that their audiences tune them out and replace them with listening to and enjoying their favorite music or learning to play a musical instrument.

I recommend that you read the lyrics and listen to the music related to each chapter before going on to the next one if possible. It will help you see how inspiring the songs are. The lyrics and music can easily be accessed from your favorite websites or through public libraries. It is hoped to have an audiobook and soundtrack produced for the visually and hearing impaired sometime after this book's publication. The audiobook and soundtrack would include the fifty lyrics and music by those artists that helped inspire this book. Figure 21-A in chapter 21 is a listing of those fifty songs and their artists.

# 1.

# Observation
# not Discrimination

I often tell people that I do not believe in discrimination but rather observation. My hope is that this point resonates with readers, chapter after chapter. That statement is probably the most important and genuine statement in this entire book. Most people I tell that to ask, "What do you mean by that?" I tell them that I practice not judging too quickly, and everyone should work at being more objective. It is okay to observe without a snap opinion. People have a right to their opinion, and their opinion in most cases is based on their social, environmental, and educational experiences. My approach to observations is based on over twenty years working in the quality assurance field. I performed products and services testing and prepared procedures in the public sector. I practiced using the scientific method when needed.

[1]A dictionary defines the *scientific method* as: the principles and procedures for a systematic pursuit of knowledge involving recognition and formulation of problems and the collection of data through observation and experimentation. For example, if I really wanted to know how many miles per gallon of gasoline my automobile achieves, I would measure the amount of gasoline used and the mileage driven, and I would compute those figures (data). Additionally, I would perform several experiments in conditions with varied outside temperature, road conditions, tire wear, etc. From this data I would form a theory (the analysis of a set of facts as they relate to one another). The figures would show a more accurate number of miles per gallon for my automobile than what the manufacturer may state.

[2]That same dictionary defines *observation* in the scientific sense as : the act of recognizing and then noting facts or occurrences, often involving measurements with instruments, and obtaining a record or description.

[3]The definition for *discrimination* is: a prejudice or prejudicial outlook, action, or treatment, or instances of discriminating categorically rather than individually.

Our country's constitution and laws state that it is illegal to practice discrimination. The Civil Rights Act of 1964 is a federal law signed by President Lyndon Johnson. It prohibits discrimination based on race, color, religion, sex, and national origin by federal and state government's public places such as schools and offices (maybe even on broadcast television or computer screens in those places). This landmark decision was made to protect all Americans from prejudicial action by organizations in the aforementioned fields. All Americans should be cognizant of this law, and all should understand the consequences should they fail to practice it and embrace it.

[4]That same dictionary defines *bigot* as 1) an obstinate or intolerant devotion to one's own opinions and prejudices. For bigotry 1) the state of mind of a bigot, 2) acts or beliefs characteristic of a bigot. Like racial bigotry. Being obstinate or intolerant is a key point. For example, if many satellite/cable news outlets and internet social media outlets colluded to throw an election toward a political candidate they were backing, and used biased, hurtful commercials, it would most probably affect the election's outcome. Continuous posting of this material days before the election could even defame the opposing candidate's character. This could be done hundreds of times in the days leading up to the election—their paid employees and associated advertising companies trying to change your opinions and beliefs about the opposing candidate. If they succeeded in swaying your beliefs with these false statements and advertising, YOU may be swayed and become a bigot.

A Russian scientist, Ivan Pavlov, studied this method of using continual cues with dogs. Today we call that method *condition response*, *conditioned emotional response,* or *condition reflex.* The Soviet Union used this method to control its people with lies for decades with their state-run propaganda newspaper *Pravda,* and it worked! Nazi Germany used similar propaganda tactics during their rise to power in the 1930s. The Nazis continued to tell their people lies, and it also worked. It was easy for these two groups, one on the extreme political left and the other on the extreme right, to continually tell lies because both were Godless socialist platforms. The internet and TV are conduits for the information received by our brains, and we use them habitually. Electronic devices are used so often they are drowning out our previous quality mentoring institutions like our parents, family members, churches, schools, and social circles.

Today, social media users often ask their followers to give "what do you think" feedback about some supposed piece of "news." Soon afterward they query their audience with pigeonholing questions. Many times those questions contain biased cues. But more importantly, the instantaneous results often do not include any truths or even worthwhile opinions and can be a paradox. This rating system, if used by our judicial system, would put a time limit on every juried case, say five minutes for the prosecution, defense, and jury to knock out a fair decision. Is that enough time to present and digest the case information and decide? The point here is that the data collected by many media groups can be flawed and slanted to support their initial intent. People need more time to gather the facts and judge adequately. It does not do any of us any good when these media news outlets present their results from this flawed system as a social conclusion. Media news is driven by how much airtime can be sold, and that is the bottom line for the networks' existence.

With our dependence on these networks, colluding media giants could purposely increase their advertising of alcohol and drugs during our nation's election campaigns to entice you to consume those products. This would obviously impair your thoughts about the elections. The impairing of Americans is the key point. Throw a few beer commercials on the five o'clock news and testosterone supplements on the ten o'clock news, and they have you hooked. I know you are asking, "Why would media employees conspire with their superiors to do this?" Simply to keep their jobs. Remember the saying, "He who pays the piper calls the tune." Also, maybe they are just stressed out in their fast-paced jobs and have a clouded view too. Some may feel that, as professional media people, they know what their audience wants to hear, even if it is not true. I believe others in the media are sitting back and watching to see if any controlling methods being used can actually affect their audience's decisions on many issues, especially elections, which may even take down a nation.

The point I'm trying to make here is to show you why we all must seek out the facts before we judge, and to understand that untruths are thrown at us all the time! It is also important to understand the difference between factual information told by reputable journalists and information that is only studio-produced entertainment. Made-for-TV entertainment provides no more factual information than the comedy shows of the day. Viewers watching "news" networks have a difficult time separating real journalistic news and what is nothing more than actors staging opinions to stimulate interest.

While growing up in the inner city, my best friend was Ronny Moore. Back then he would have been known as "colored." Today, I guess (for now), he is labeled African-American. For me, my friend was not colored, a negro, a Black person, or an African-American, but only my best friend. One day after school I stopped over at Ronny's house. He lived on Trumbull Avenue, right behind the public school we attended. For me this was cool because my dad grew up on Trumbull Avenue, just a few houses from Ronny's. I met Ronny's mom and grandmother, and they greeted me with kindness. To them I was just one of Ronny's third-grade friends. As kids we did things that eight-year-olds did. We rode bikes and played baseball on the playgrounds. Maybe we made a little mischief like breaking a window in an abandoned house (hey, half the windows were already broken). Jimmy Stewart and Donna Reed did that in the movie *It's a Wonderful Life*. Sometimes I guess kids just imitate what they view on TV. The point here is that my friendship with Ronny was real, and our parents observed and approved of it. I will never forget the time I invited him to my third-grade after-school religion class at St. Wenceslaus Church. When he got into the classroom he looked around and took it all in. My teacher was a nun and had me introduce him to the class. Hey, I was a kid in an integrated school before forced busing, and it was all okay. I think maybe that is when my parents figured I might grow up to be a problem for them.

I had another friend that lived behind our corner house in Cleveland. He lived on Victor Avenue. His name was Johnny Cloud. He told me he was part Indian (Native American or whatever) and asked me if I wanted to be a blood brother. At nine years old that was cool. So, he pulled out this switch blade and cut a mark in his right hand and mine, and we tightly shook hands. What are friends for? I guess the kids in my neighborhood did not have dual Roy Rogers six-shooters like mine, so they carried knives. I learned later to never bring a toy gun to a knife fight.

Another friend from my school was named Juan. We rode our bikes together. One day we pulled into Juan's yard on Nursery Street, and his eight-year-old brother Valentino walked out on his front porch. I guess his mother told him to protect the house until Juan came home. Anyway, Valentino came out with this knife, and he cut me above my wrist. I still have the scar. If it were not for Juan stopping him, the crazy kid would probably have killed me. Today we are worried about gun control—hell, what about knife control?

It was different for me to think about color issues until the riots in the 1960s. The interesting thing about the riots was that they mostly happened after the 1964 Civil Rights Act. Logically you would think the riots would have led to that landmark act. Some people may have interpreted the Civil Rights Act as *enabling* the riots. Later I learned that the riots were mostly caused by historical and geographical reasons. Many children and grandchildren of the southern slaves moved north and west looking for better opportunities for work and a better life. Because of the racial bigotry existing in the South at that time (not necessarily today), a white phobia developed in those families and was carried to their new homes. Believe me, this feeling they held is understandable and justified, period. Deep cuts are long to heal. For people in the North, like my parents, if you used the word *boy* it meant "young male." To these new residents it was derogatory. The term *white phobia* is not meant to be derogatory, but to categorize a social issue that exists to this day and is still dismissed. For descendants of southern slaves, dismissing this fear is similar to what John Wayne said in one of his movies, if you replace "sorry" with "afraid": "Never say you're sorry, it's a sign of weakness." Due to oppression from Southerners, descendants of the slaves acquired a natural prejudice against most white people and needed to build their self-esteem and act in self-preservation. It is much like looking at a lion or tiger right in their eyes.

An especially important question for all Americans is: Are we living in a white man's society in the United States? I did not give any amount of thought to that at one time. However, I am sure that we are not, and here is why. Americans elected Barak Obama as President of the United States—the highest position in our country—twice. Make no mistake, Barak Obama is not only a minority, he is a mix of races, and of a Muslim background. Also, an important fact relative to culture, our founding fathers were being abused by the British, which started the American Revolution. It did not matter if the folks in the thirteen colonies were of any particular race. Great Britain, as a monarchy, chartered a company, the West Indies Company, to increase their commerce, and was prepared to rule the waves and the world at any cost or loss of life. For Great Britain, this goal was like our space race during the 1960s. Some powerful nations today may be trying to emulate what Great Britain did over two centuries ago.

In the 1700s the North had some industries, and the South had plantations. The British government began enabling the entrepreneur colonists in the new world, supplying whatever it took to produce goods, then demanded that the colonists pay outrageously high taxes. *Slavery became an enabling act.* Any good Christian, Jew, Hindu, Buddhist, or Muslim with any religious consciousness or compassion would never have allowed this practice. However, that old devil's ideology and man's selfishness said, "If it's good for me to make money and grow the economy, and there is no law against it, it must be good for all." That darn devil. Correct, there was no law, but the truth of the matter is that it was mostly good for the British government and their contractors. I see a trend in the world today as it was back then.

After the Revolutionary War, our forefathers drafted a government that was as fair and as flexible as it could be. There were guaranteed rights and mechanisms in place to make it the best and most democratic government possible. As for slavery, it took a civil war to eradicate it; a war caused by southern politicians backed by affluent plantation owners, who convinced poorer working folks to fight for them. It almost sounds like a similar situation we have with big-money groups trying to influence young people to riot and tear down our cities, as was done during the pandemic. However, as the song goes, "The truth marches on." Slavery in this country is dead, period, unless you want to become slaves to a controlling government.

The next humanitarian issue to die in this country should be all forms of bigotry, hate, or personal gain from special interest groups and lobbyists. As a democracy we are supposed to be the controlling force against those actions like the skewed version of diversity, which does not contain strict, fair parameters for all Americans and is clouding everyone's understanding of human rights, culture, free thought, liberty, and most importantly respect for *everyone.*

I never ran a race I did not think I could win. That is what happens when you play tag on a playground with kids that are as fast as lightning.

I will make my point. I am a male, and it states that on my birth certificate. I am proud of that fact. *Viva la difference!* Also listed are hair and eye color, and that is really the only things that need to be listed. As Americans and God's children, we are all created equal. I feel I am a person of color. For me, if you would call me white, I would consider that as offensive as if you called me "pale face." If you must call me any color, race, or background, call me "neutral." Unlike some people in our country, I do not have an identity problem. I do not need to be called brown, red, yellow, black, African-American, or Hispanic for exploitation or political purposes. Being of a scientific nature I often witness how statistics can be used and misused. I think it is time to end the use of race or gender in any job application, college entrance application, or for any purpose. Inquiring about any American's personal background for documenting purposes is, by itself, an act of discrimination. From my observations the inquiry into one's biological makeup is the main cause for racial discord in our country today and should be abolished. All too often our politicians today prey on identity groups for their election purposes as opposed to addressing the social issues facing us. Their shell game and diversionary tactics only divide our nation's ability to unify us for the common good and to resolve our identified problems. Americans put themselves in a racial pickle when they started to differentiate our people for military service or government jobs based on racial identity. That action was a big mistake and must be undone, but try un-ringing a bell. Martin Luther King stated that people should be judged by their character and not by the color of their skin.

For this chapter, my inspiration came from the song "Break on Through." It was written and performed by the rock group the Doors. I really believe people must break through their possible brainwashed thinking from news outlets, social media, and TV advertisements today, and their appetite for sports, entertainment, libations, and drugs, and strive to get the facts. Many people need to get the facts about bigotry and discrimination, to talk about them and not harbor any predetermined thoughts about them. Unfortunately, that takes time, *but you must take that time*. You must develop a strong self-discipline and be objective. Your need to vote on important issues and not identity politics. We need to get our minds and bodies right and get straight! In chapter 17, "Government, Economics, Politics and Defense" I will discuss the three sides of politics that are triangular, not linear, as most have been taught. Politics are not just a "left" and "right" thing. There is a third side, the one I hope you will break on through to.

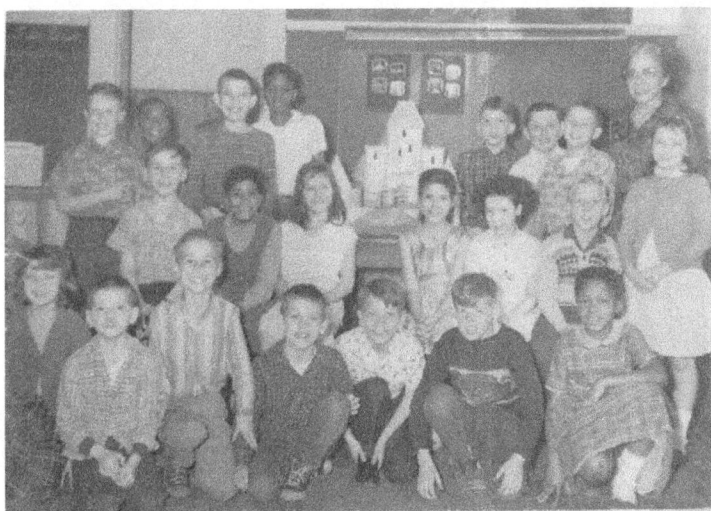

*This photo is of Mrs. Wilkins's third-grade class and was taken by her husband. I'm in the middle row, sixth from the left. My best friend, Ronny Moore, is in the top row, fourth from the left.*

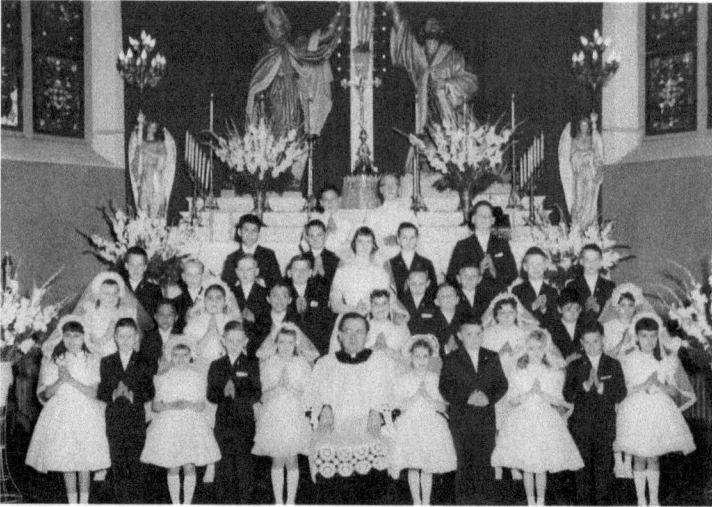

*This is my First Communion photo from St. Wenceslaus Church in 1961. I attended public school religion classes for this ceremony. My friend Ronny Moore attended one of those classes with me. I'm in row three, second from the left.*

# 2.

# Rights and the Right Thing to Do (Acts of Kindness)

The first time I thought about rights and the right thing to do was when our neighbor's twelve-year-old son crossed in front of my family-filled van on our little two-lane road. He didn't just cross, he sauntered across the road, taking his good old time. I was a little agitated by this because I made it a practice to hurry across any road, street, avenue, or whatever before I got ran over. My wife calmly explained to me that "he had the right to cross the street." I got that, but I responded, "Walking extremely slow...it's just not the right thing to do. You can get injured, and what about respect for the car's driver?" My wife explained that the boy did that to agitate me and express his rights. It was a good thing that my brakes were working properly. The other point here is that he was being disrespectful, law or no law, and it was still a borderline hateful act. An act of kindness would have been for the neighbor boy to stop and wave me on (there was not a crosswalk on the road). Acts of kindness toward others outside of our families help to cement our culture and values.

Before that neighborhood encounter I really never gave much thought about the difference between rights and the right thing to do. It is not usually a household discussion. In one of my college management classes our professor asked the class, "What is more important: to do things right, or to do the right things?" If you do something, anything in business or in life, that action can either be the right thing to do or the wrong thing. Doing wrong things correctly can be a waste of time and money. Therefore, the answer is—ding, ding, ding—doing the right things! Yes, there are alternatives. However, the question is, are you *mostly* doing the right things? The best things?

Taking a minute to think about our rights, I am reminded of our inalienable rights stated by Thomas Jefferson in our Declaration of Independence. These rights are guaranteed by our Constitution. However, by my observations, we take our rights way too much for granted. So much so that many times we think we have the freedom to do almost anything. However, having those rights and practicing doing the right things are different concepts and actions.

Going back further, our beloved pilgrims fled England 150 years before our Revolutionary War to find freedom from religious persecution in England. Later, Americans revolted against British tyranny and fought for our independence to create a new nation with a better system. This was done primarily because of a not righteous leader, King George, and the unscrupulous terms of the British trading companies. The people back then, even living with a system of laws, did not do the right things toward their fellow man.

I always presume people strive to do the right things. Again, we take our rights for granted. Where this whole issue becomes complex is when you try to scientifically measure the differences between rights and the right things to do. In a legal sense, any lawyer would advise you to follow all laws, and you should be okay. However, what if there were no laws to cover certain actions? As a famous cartoon cricket says, always let your conscience be your guide. Ask yourself if you are practicing doing the *right* things. Are your actions based on financial gain, pleasure, or your character? Will your decisions be purely selfish acts or benefit others as well?

Since I became aware of the difference between rights and the right things to do, I have observed a few things. When I was the quality assurance guru on my job, I had a situation where our caulking guns were not working. We purchased many of these caulking guns from a small company in northeast Ohio. So, I placed a phone call to that supplier. This was when companies actually had people that answered phone calls because *they actually cared* what their customers' concerns were! I explained to the administrator that the caulking guns supplied to us did not work. Her question to me was, how much did you pay for them? I told her they were $3.55 each. With that she told me I should have expected failures when we paid only $3.55 for caulking guns. I said, "I expected them to work!" They took them back and credited our account. The point here is, first, the guns should not have been poorly manufactured, and second, the person handling the items for return should have been more professional about it. She had the right to tell me what her attitude was about the price of the guns; however, professionally it was not the right thing to do. Whatever happened to the sayings "the customer is always right" or "the customer is king"?

In a similar situation, my wife's carpenter uncle, Danny, from Altoona, Pennsylvania, was helping me put a roof on our home's addition. He was up at the top of the house, nailing the pieces of hip-roof rafters that I had to cut. These pieces of lumber had tricky angle cuts, not only across the face of the wood but also angled across the edge. After three failed cuts I apologized and said I would get it right the next time. With that he said, "It really doesn't matter to me. I can't see this problem all the way from Altoona!"

My uncle's comment about the distance from his home and the failed caulking guns gave me an epiphany of what is going on with all these poorly made products we are purchasing from China. These products have an unbelievably high failure rate because they are made for internet pricing only. If their products do not work, it wastes our time and our money. The companies that sell these failed products do not return them to China, because the shipping costs would be prohibitive. *Most of them end up in our landfills.* I can visualize the Chinese sellers on the other end of the telephone discussing these failures and saying, "I do not see your problem with that product all the way from here in Beijing." It is another way of saying, with all the remote workforces out there, "Out of site and out of mind!" That is something for consumers to consider about the quality of their purchases. *Buyers do need to know up front where their products are made.*

I am going to end this shoddy products example with the most ridiculous one. How many times have you seen these one-minute commercials on late-night television about wonder drugs? They advertise these medical products to hopefully help sufferers with their pain or afflictions. The disclaimer for those products, due to their aftereffects, take up more than thirty seconds of the one-minute commercial. It is no wonder why people just do not understand this dysfunctional society we are living in. God help us so that the world's governments finally do the right things and not just do things because they have the right. They should take the time to test products and stop having the general public be the guinea pigs for them. *Drugs that may prove to be if harmful to the public should be banned completely!*

In the previous paragraph I said that our society is becoming "dysfunctional." I am going to scientifically explain that theory and how it relates to rights and the right thing to do. [1]A dictionary states that something *functional* is 2) used to contribute to the development or maintenance of a larger whole, and is designed or developed chiefly from the point of view of use. Simply put, functionality indicates things are working in harmony together, whether it is devices or, on a larger scale, societies. [2]*Dysfunction* is defined as :impaired or abnormal functioning. It is abnormal or unhealthy interpersonal behavior or interaction within a group. "Impaired" is a key point and will be discussed later in chapter 7, "Our Drugged Society."

My wife and I are very family-oriented people. Family will be discussed in more detail in a later chapter too. However, because of our love for our children we became involved in Cub Scouts, then Boy Scout and Girl Scouts. These organizations have been and still are exceptionally good character-building programs for children and young adults. I was and still am a volunteer in Scouting programs. Both organizations have guidelines and principles which their participants follow. [3]In scouting, their motto is to "be prepared." Being prepared is functional; being unprepared, as it relates to group reliance, is dysfunctional. The Scouts practice an oath. [4]The Boy Scout Oath states to do duty to God and country and to obey the scout law. [5]The Scout Law has twelve points. They are to be trustworthy, loyal, helpful, friendly, courteous, kind, obedient, cheerful, thrifty, brave, clean, and reverent.

Let us act out a case and do a 180-degree difference, a mathematical reciprocal or reverse of these guidelines. Let us NOT do duty to God, NOT do duty to country, and NOT obey the Scout Law. I think you are starting to understand my point. Place an *un-* in front of each of the Scout Laws and try living them. These laws sound like good advice for a society to build upon. Having a society that does the reverse of these Scout Laws would be problematic. If people did the reverse of these guidelines because they have their rights, they would follow no guidelines, purposely, even rebelliously, to get their way. However, these people have no clear directional heading, like a compass with a continually spinning magnetic needle unable to point north. They are just hoping their elected leaders will lead them and forgetting that the political candidates will tell them anything to get elected. Especially when it comes to making them feel good and not asking them for their time or money.

The scouting point was only one example of the difference between rights and the right things to do. Let us use an example of a precept from one world religion. [6]Consider the Ten Commandments:

1. I am the Lord your God, who brought you out of the land of Egypt: You shall not have other gods beside me.
2. You shall not invoke the name of the Lord, your God, in vain (wicked, worthless, or no good purpose).

3. Remember the sabbath day-keep it holy.
4. Honor thy father and your mother, that you may have a long life in the land the Lord your God has given you.
5. You shall not kill.
6. You shall not commit adultery.
7. You shall not commit steal.
8. You shall not bear false witness against your neighbor.
9. You shall not covet your neighbor's house.
10. You shall not covet your neighbor's wife , his male or female slave, his ox or donkey, or anything that belongs to your neighbor.

Let us look at the reverse of these religious principles. To specifically not follow these principles and act against them would be…again, you fill in the blank! If a person lived in a society that fostered these reverse principles, frustration and hate could easily develop. At our house we taught our children never to use the word *hate*. What type of Godless society might this be? Living in a society as described would be dangerous *and*, *yes*, dysfunctional.

I would like to go back to my point about putting an un- before known functions that are proven to work and could be labeled the "right things to do." Suppose if some group with organizational skills had an agenda to make America a greater society, and they used logical and practical methods. Through factual data, they achieved those goals and showed social and economic improvements (growth). Couldn't those results be construed as the "right things to do"? For a reversal of those positive results, place an un- in front of each. How would you feel if another group replaced that functional group's results instantaneously and un-did all of the functional improvements that were achieved. It could therefore be construed that this new group purposely made America less functional and worked in the direction of creating a dysfunctional society. My point is made. Why would this group do that? It certainly goes against logic!

Perhaps a revolution without firing a shot? Maybe even worse than that, weakening our nation and leaving our gates open.

It is easy to see from these examples that many of these social guidelines go along the lines of morality. I knew someone that was a big pornographic magazine guy. He said to me countless times that you can't legislate morality. I told him that I do not wish to legislate morality. I just would like to live in a system, country, or world where my family is safe from theft, murder, drugs, envy, vanity, and Godlessness.

As previously pointed out, you can do the right things, or, whether you choose to believe it or not, do the wrong things! In many instances there are gray areas between the two. However, if you use what is called English logic, it helps one to make choices between those decisions. English logic follows three simple principles. They are information, decision, and action. The information part is the most important. You must have good, honest resources to provide verifiable information. Then take the time to analyze them. Then choose your right decisions from a few selected choices (a few choices are always good things), and then act. In situations where someone can be bombarded with information, one should use what is called Occam's razor. In this process the simplest explanation is usually correct. This process "shaves" away the least likely outcome.

For this chapter, my inspiration came from the song "For What It's Worth." It was written by Steven Stills and performed by the rock group Buffalo Springfield. If you know anything about the history of the song, regardless of the lyrics, it was considered a big Vietnam War protest song of the 1960s. This song epitomizes where rights and the right thing to do come together. America was involved in a senseless war. There were thousands of young American servicepeople dying in that war, and for what? Most people did not care for a seemingly endless war, and most other countries did not want us there. In the height of this war, four protesting students died on the Kent State campus (which is my two daughters' alma mater). That shooting happened two years *after* the song "For What It's

Worth" was released. However, it is not often that rights and the right thing to do are called into action. If you see something or, more importantly, you know the truth about something, and it is not RIGHT, you have the tools to fix it: vote.

# 3.

# Your Character, Our Country, and Our Culture

This chapter's intent is to provide awareness of your personal habits and is a preview of the next few chapters. Your habits may be limiting your ability to perform at peak levels. We are referring to both your mental and physical levels. A healthy YOU better assures that your family and friends see that you are taking care of yourself, which in turn may allow you to take better care of them. It is cheap insurance that says you are also trying not to potentially be a physical or mental burden on them. A healthier you also strengthens our country. You do play a large role in safeguarding our liberties and freedoms. You do vote, don't you? We will discuss your personal limiting habits that affect your performance. They are:

1. The amount of alcohol that you drink. What is the difference between social drinking intolerance and outright alcoholism?
2. The amount of drugs you take, whether prescription or non-prescription. This includes smoking or vaping.
3. The amount of time spent on traditional entertainment.
4. The amount of time and money you spend on vanity entertainment like gaming, fantasy sports, or gambling.
5. The amount of time you spend listening to and interacting on social media.
6. The type of food you eat. Much like those computer classes you were required to take, garbage in equates to garbage out!
7. Any indifference or even ignorance by you to improve your

well-being. Are you any type of caring person, even the type that will not care for yourself?

An inventory of your habits is necessary to determine where you are now and to put you on a path to understand that this road you are on is shared by other travelers. Putting up a *get out of my way* sign will only lead you to a crash, or road rage with others wearing the same signs. The highway ramp we are trying to put you on is not Interstate "I one," but rather a roundabout with little congestion and a safe way home. Your safe way home begins with you enacting a program of self-discipline and eliminating poor social habits.

You would hope that everyone's goal in his or her pursuit of happiness would be to become an able and productive member of our society. There is nothing better than everyone paying their fair share of taxes, and in the process *lowering* yours. My wife always says, "laziness trumps everything." In Thomas Jefferson's own words, he said you have the rights to life, liberty, and the pursuit of happiness. Hopefully, your neighbor is not some anarchist with an agenda to derail your life's vision, nor the one Thomas Jefferson had.

In your pursuit of happiness, are you taking care of yourself physically and mentally? It is difficult to be productive if you are not the best you can be. It is encouraging today to see many of our cities providing recreational facilities for their residents. Remember though, it is not about you alone. What are you doing to help other people? Maybe you can positively affect that anarchist neighbor who has probably been brainwashed by social media, and get him or her to see the light. It may be trite, but we are all in this thing together.

President John F. Kennedy said in his inaugural address, "Ask not what your country can do for you—ask what you can do for your country." That is a great credo to follow. I do not believe he was referring to the geographical country, but we the people, one. I can remember being in grade school, and we followed what was then called the Presidential Physical Fitness Award Program. With the obesity problem children are facing today, it may not be such a bad idea to get that program going again and maybe even kick it up a notch.

The obesity issue could also be attributed to many factors. One obvious factor was our move from a manufacturing-based nation to a service-based one, which began in the 1990s. Restaurants and fast-food outlets have skyrocketed since then. That is an example of a cause-effect cycle. More specifically, it takes two incomes to support a household because of the lack of higher paying trade or union jobs in general. Both parents are in the daily workforce and too exhausted to cook a meal at the family table, which necessitates fast food for dinner. In retrospect, families used to gather at the quiet dinner table while looking at each other, and *they discussed important issues* that may have affected their family. Just think: no steering wheel in the way, no cell phone in the face or Bluetooth device blaring a conversation with someone that no one cares about. At *your* family table there should be a tablecloth draped over it with the words, *This is what God intended REAL quality time to mean.* These are your habits, your routines, and how they affect you and your family.

If we can ever get our big industrial machine cranked up and going again, our world's adversaries will wonder what caused this great transformation. A newer approach to American manufacturing will be discussed in our last chapter. The EPA's help in improving and developing more ecofriendly modern production methods will make for happier workforces and an appreciation of how we feel about each other's well-being and about having less stress in the workplace. Hopefully, it will lead to using less unhealthy habits like cigarettes, vaping, beer, wine, recreational marijuana, or opioids. Spending time working out or even running, biking, or hiking takes us away from some nonproductive habitual activities like watching our large-screen TVs or habitually using our many other electronic devices today. It seems like when we are using those aforementioned

31

devices we *cannot* get away from these pesky, time-consuming and alluring advertisements. Many of those alluring advertisements are about drinking more alcohol, eating more junk food, and gaining more weight. Thank God they don't show smoking products on TV today. Please realize that the advertiser's products are there for them and their business partners' monetary benefit, and not necessarily for *your* benefit. A cycle of watching TV and being on the internet without a routine of exercise may lead to depression or other health problems. Depression may lead to alcohol or drug abuse. Your health is important to all of us because your bad habits can be costly for all of us. Keep yourself as physically active as you safely can, and keep your mind free of *impairments*, such as alcohol or drug abuse. Concentrate on things that can make a positive influence on your family and friends. Use your energy by donating it to groups that are physically, mentally, or *legitimately* economically disadvantaged.

I did not mention it in this book's preface, but I am a big professional sports fan. As a kid from Cleveland, I enjoy watching the Cleveland Guardians (formally the Indians), Browns, and Cavaliers as much as I can. I can recall Marty Schottenheimer, a former Cleveland Browns head coach, once saying that you only get out of anything that which you put into it. He was a great coach and often gave motivational speeches to his team. Another one of his sayings was, you play as you practice. Many times, high-profile sports figures forget that they are playing on a TEAM sport. The point here is, *we* are playing on a team sport every day. Just like the sports figures that get caught up in their agent's hype about their value, we get caught up with those same personal ego problems and lose sight of the team's goals for winning. It is not always about the money. Like we have heard many times, money cannot buy everything. I have heard from many elderly people in my business that if you have your health, you have everything. I really believe there is no substitute for experience, and the elderly have it.

The word *culture* gets thrown around too often today by everyone and used as an excuse for all our present social problems. There are two basic dictionary definitions for the word *culture*. Paraphrasing, the first is the customary beliefs, social forms, and material traits of a social group. This definition is what I have observed and term to be the *excuses* or *results* definition. The second definition is an acquaintance with and taste in arts, humanities, and science as distinguished from vocational and technical skills. This definition is the creative one for a culture. The latter *embellishes* the former. The latter definition is the dog wagging its tail instead of the tail wagging the dog. Isn't the latter definition the one that should define you and your country? This is the one you can proudly say you contributed to, with your name on it, and no one can take your fine deeds away from it. Every day you are a working part of our American culture to make it a model for all to follow and aspire to. It starts with *you*, and you can make the difference. A mentor of mine once told me the roads to Rome were not paved by good intentions. Do not just talk about your ideas and values, *do something about them.*

For this chapter, the music that inspired me to write it came from the song "Something Good." It was written by Richard Rodgers and sung by Julie Andrews and Christopher Plummer as a duet in *The Sound of Music*. It is one of my favorite movies. It captures many of the topics discussed in this book and some of my observations. Its themes are religion, family, romance, and of course music. It is about the family von Trapp of Austria, and how the crazy Nazis in the 1930s affected their family by forcing an invading government's will on them. The most important message taken from the song "Something Good" is that nothing comes from nothing, and nothing ever can. That is the essence of this chapter. It is about *your character, your country and our culture.* You must, as the old US Army recruiting advertisements used to say, be the best that you can be! We need you to help get this ship, our country, headed on a course of sustained prosperity. No one person or group can do it alone. Let us get the synergy flowing and get your engine started without high-energy drinks. Eat a healthy diet from the three main food groups. Have a daily exercise program and get at least six to seven hours of sleep every night (consecutively). This ship needs a healthy crew of strong bodies and minds. Dr. Phil and Dr. Oz are not out there for you to sit in front of your TV screen munching on highly seasoned taco chips, wishing you could help. Turn off the television and start contributing with a sound mind and body.

# 4.

# Selfishness and Vanity

There is no word in the English language that hits the mark better than the word self. How precise that word is. An even more precise word is when you add the – ish to selfish. In this chapter, I will discuss today's emphasis on the increasing amount of selfishness and vanity in America today. [1]A dictionary defines selfish as: 1) concerned excessively or exclusively with oneself: seeking or concentrating on one's own advantage, pleasure, or well-being without regard for others. There is an old saying that goes, they can't see the forest for the trees. In this case your own self is in the way of you being able to have an unbiased interaction with others and tapping your own potential as a human or, better put, a humane being.

In the preface I talked about the dichotomy between the twentieth and twenty-first centuries. Comparatively speaking, this twenty-first century most definitely reeks of human selfishness. In a previous chapter I referred to this century as "the century of self-fulfilling prophecies." I have lived in this century over twenty years now and can attest that Americans today, as opposed to the past, are living and smirking with an overwhelming amount of human selfishness. People today are so self-centered on getting their own way it becomes all-consuming for them. For those with some power and influence, especially in government or industry, they will drop whatever their immediate responsibilities are to achieve their selfishness.

Another example of selfishness today is where employees at work (or working from their home) tend to do their personal activities on their company's time. Where are a person's ethics to do this? With the advent of smartphones, employees are looking for any excuse at work to get on their phones and text someone about God only knows what. The real kicker is where employees, 1) either use their company's computers to buy online items or, 2) just pick up their smartphones and do it all on their company's time. For the cool employers it is called a loss of productivity, the employees' waste of time, and is costly not only for their firm but collectively to our nation. When these cool employers make out their labor budgets, they should keep that in mind. Maybe they are getting free pandemic money for this insanity.

My parents, and the parents of their generation, raised us with the goal of making sure that their children had a better life then they had. For them, their world happened during our Great Depression. Even without considering that catastrophe, don't *you* want your children to be more successful than you? I am talking about your children holistically. I'm referring to their mind, body, disposition, and hell, their very soul! These children are not your pets; they are more than just objects. *They are the future of the world.*

My parents and others strived to make sure our nation would become a better, stronger, and safer one. What a noble goal. Black or white, richer or poorer, these folks were self-sacrificing, goal-oriented, and tenacious. What am I looking at today? What do I see others doing? I see people being hypnotized by their smartphones. Their eyes are glued to those phones. Please, if you can, lift your eyes up from your phone and look around you. Do you see how you have been locked to your smartphone screen (or large TV screen) lately? I propose we replace these phones with three-by-five mirrors that have built-in timers that go off every hour during the day. Just think of it: We no longer would be paying those high-priced cell phone bills. While looking in that mirror, you'd take account of some of your recent selfish actions. Who recently have you hurt with these actions? What have you said or done that benefited others? Social media only tells you what your little selfish mind wants to hear anyway. Even calling them cell "phones" is a misnomer. In reality they have become more like miniature Chinese billboards: "sell" phones. They continually are blinking advertisements for big sales of yoga pants or for whatever—only God knows. Emotional response to them only generates artificial intelligence, and is only emotionally based.

In chapter 2 we tried to simplify decisions as being the right decisions or the wrong ones. Of course, there are gray areas in that process, not just black and white, and *a few options are always a good thing*. While I am on the subject of human selfishness, let us say there are two kinds of people, introverts and extroverts, even though many agree there are five basic categories. They are: extroversion (assertiveness), agreeableness (social affection), openness (insight/imagination), conscientiousness (detailed organizers), and neuroticism (moody). The one group, extroverts, typically are vying for attention. The other groups can either be indifferent to attention or *avoid it*. Yes, that is a big generalization, but look at the obvious signs. Consider, for example, tattoos. Would you say that people who display their tattoos have a self-esteem issue? In many cases it is their artful expression. How about today's emphasis on fashion? What is with the big attraction to being mainstream today anyway? Is it the extrovert in you displaying your appetite for attention, or is it that you want to be cool just like your friends? Are they really your friends, or are they your competition? You may not live up to their cool high standards, and they have no problem telling you about it or, better still, talking behind your back about it. Whether it is clothing or the building of one's peer group (gangs), there is little time for your mental solitude and well-being. You need to take a few moments for a much-needed self-evaluation. For most people, before they go to sleep, they usually think about things they did during the day and the next day's schedule. Before falling asleep, have that first thought be about the deed you did that day and how it benefited a needy person. Maybe you need to at least say a prayer for them. Please, take a moment and take an account of your "self."

Whatever happened to the Mother Teresas of this world? She was born in Macedonia, north of Greece. She was a Catholic nun and dedicated her entire life to helping other people. For that she is now titled Saint Teresa of Calcutta. I recently saw an example of these Mother Teresas as they took care of my mother and many others in her nursing home before she died in 2019. These tireless people, almost all considering themselves women of color today, took unbelievable care of my mother in her final days and hours. I am observing an untapped resource of people today that are lost in a life of misdirection, looking for a purpose other than a life of despair they feel they are bound to. I know there is a college debt crisis. I only hope that the debt owed isn't affecting people to doubt the positions they have obtained so far. I see a possible army of folks able to turn *their* world around and make *our* world brighter. We will discuss a proposal that may turn your future and our nation around in this book's last chapter.

We do *not* need cities of despair, as Calcutta was. Look at our big cities today. The mess created by political ideology aimed at the destruction of those cities by labeling them 'sanctuary cities' has created a need and opportunity to help the needy. Groups like churches and others should help to get these people out of those cities and into facilities that can house, feed, and clothe them, and help them get righted into a life of prosperity instead of despair. Please, if you have the capacity, volunteer and be that Mother Teresa, Father Flannigan, or Father Damien. Father Flannigan was an Irish-born priest. He founded the orphanage for troubled youths known as Boys Town, which is in Boys Town, Nebraska. Father Damien was a Belgian priest. He is recognized for his ministry in the Kingdom of Hawaii. He helped people with leprosy in the nineteenth century.

I mentioned that our children are this country's future. That is a fact, and we need to establish that as a baseline in our country's educational system. Over the past several years there has been an emphasis on building our children's self-esteem, both in our homes and especially in our schools. There may be a self-esteem issue for some school children but not all of them. For the children that do not have self-esteem issues, they see the over-encouragement as being a foolish waste of their time. Every student should be recognized for their work and continually encouraged to do their best, but give the encouragement to the ones that need it most.

Where is the safety net for our children to prevent acts of selfishness? Our children experience the all-alluring, almost bewitching realm of social media and electronic devices that alter their ability to make unbiased decisions. We keep hearing about children being abducted by strangers they met through the internet, but as a society we do not press the issue to prevent it. Big Tech's disclaimer for their responsibilities is, "You opened the page, didn't you." Big Tech *made our society dependent on their devices* so we could make our society better—or was it to satisfy our vanity or selfishness or just make more money for *them and their business manufacturing partners*? You will have to ponder that one for a while before you decide on it.

Our youth, and this includes many of their parents, have been taught that their expectations for success are to exceed those of their neighbors. What happened to those good neighbors that were your friends that you could count on? Have you turned them into your competition? There is an old saying: They are just keeping up with the Joneses. These days people smirk as they try to pass anyone up on their all-important measuring stick for their success. Mr. Rogers, from the popular children's TV program, is probably turning over in his grave at how you treat your neighbors. Make no mistake, selfishness and vanity go together like a horse and a carriage. We must help each other as neighbors when needed. Did Thomas Edison create the light bulb for his success or for better lighting that was needed for humanity?

Many feel that this nation is becoming a nation of spoiled little brats that are becoming more and more influenced by their face in their cell phones on one hand and their cup of brand-name coffee in the other. While doing this they are ignoring the signs of the less fortunate in need.

Get a healthy mind and body and give them a helping hand. Change some of these bad personal habits of TV watching and cell phone use. There are over four hundred national parks alone in the United States. Get out there and see some of them. Get some oxygen in your lungs and some greenery in your eyes instead of that little limelight screen or your fifty-plus-inch TV. Take a train, bus, or car ride to some historical site. Real people created these parks with their hands and not with a keyboard. You are becoming a deadhead and, even worse, a guinea pig piece of data for social media's manipulations of you. Here, push this button ( + ) if you agree with me! Nobody cares what your deadhead thinks or what your biased, selfish, brainwashed thoughts really mean. I care about your thoughts and deeds, and the people that really need your help care about them too.

The music that inspired me for this chapter came from the songs "I Want To Talk About Me," sung by Toby Keith and written by Bobby Braddock, and "You're So Vain," both sung and written by Carly E. Simon. Toby Keith gives a never-ending list of things that his girlfriend wants to talk about, but says it's *his turn* to be heard now. Carly Simon must have had some relationships with some really vain people in her life. In "You're So Vain," she describes just about the most self-centered individual on our planet. Her date is so vain that he cannot pass up a mirror without looking at himself. Mirrors do have a way of making people notice themselves, don't they? If you get anything out of this chapter please understand that the world we live in is NOT JUST ABOUT YOU!

# 5.

# Mass Media, Social Media, and Multimedia Intelligence

I have had the opportunity to visit one of central Florida's major amusement complexes a few times. It has one theme park that has many educational attractions. When I think of it, it always brings a smile to my face. There is one attraction that has an American historical significance. It is in a theater-like setting for the show. In one segment of the show they have robotic humans named Ben and Mark discussing the United States' past and how America helped shape the world for true democracy. Ben is an American political icon from the 1776 period. Mark is a famous author from the nineteenth century. The show opens with Ben discussing how it took so many times for Thomas Jefferson to complete the writing of the Declaration of Independence. Together the duo discusses the many strengths of our democratic government and the United States' accomplishments through the years. At one point Ben mentions to Mark that America is an example of a great experiment in democracy. He hit that one right on the nose. *It is an ongoing experiment.* Many from other countries and even our own home-grown citizens and visitors continually test our God-given democracy's birthright and, more importantly, its endurance.

One American experiment that has "gone wild" was the creation of the internet in the 1980s. The internet is being discussed in this chapter because it plays a very large part in all of the world's media today. It coincidentally seems to reach almost everyone with the rise of smartphone use. It has even led Big Tech corporations to exploit users' thought processes. Most users are all in lock step with the practice of using the internet automatically or even instinctively…continuously. Unfortunately, the internet was created in a similar fashion to what is called a fast-track project. Sometimes these projects occur because an organization or a person wants to take credit for it in their time. However, the management of these projects is driven by the earliest presentation date possible rather than by their quality or even their original function. This happens by ignoring the amount of time it takes to do the necessary research and testing to assure a project is safe. If they do not do enough testing it may create more problems, costs, or fallout than the project or operation itself.

We may use the analogy of the atom bomb as an example. The nuclear fallout from the radioactive dust from an atomic weapon may be worse than the bomb itself. Case in point, our withdrawal of all US troops and *some* equipment from Afghanistan a week before the twentieth anniversary of 9/11 was an example of a fast-track project. The planning, testing, and evaluations from a team of experienced personnel is critical for a high-profile project of that magnitude. Yes, we left Afghanistan after it appeared fruitless, as in South Vietnam. The difference is, there must have been a written withdrawal plan that was created and used when we left Vietnam. Many of the strategies, methods, and overall objectives should have been studied and implemented for withdrawal from Afghanistan.

This also applies to the creation of the internet. Let us face the facts: The internet has flaws. The costs that customers pay for cleanup and upkeep is proof of those flaws. These flaws are the viruses and necessary security protections against identity theft and invading harmful software. Without constant maintenance costs for virus protection, the internet itself can damage *your equipment*. The manufacturers' constant upgrades to your system or device still *never* make the internet "clinical," that is very exact, clean and secure. The internet flaws return every month as a bill, not to mention the costs for access. The internet is basically a one-channel monopoly. It is like having only one channel or station to have access to, and it is not free. Do our computers offer other "net" systems to navigate, or is there just one button on them dedicated only to connect or disconnect "the internet"?

Before the special prepaid radio and cable TV, all television and radio came into our homes or automobiles free of cost, after a one-time purchase of the TV by the consumer. This was a fact that your parents or grandparents may not have told you. In the 1970s, when television was free, there were wine commercials featuring actor-director Orson Welles as the product's spokesperson. The commercial was played often, and he said, "We will sell no wine before its time." What he was alluding to was that the wine they made would never be marketed for sale until it completed its aging process. I was in the quality assurance field for twenty-five years, and that statement says it all. Who wants watered-down wine! That statement could also apply to what is *wrong with the internet* that everyone has accepted as functioning properly.

Let's compare its functioning to that of our automobiles. It would be the same as not being able to drive our purchased cars until we paid a toll at the end of our driveways. I suppose if this were only a local city problem we could always move out from that stupid city into another. In the internet's case, there are no other "nets" to drive to. Let's continue with this example. After we pay our tolls to drive our cars, are the roads smooth? The monopolized road or cyberspace we are driving on has muggers and car thieves on it. So the correction is to pay for "mob protection" so our vehicles do not get wrecked or stolen. Hell, it would be like opening your car door and finding thieves inside it! I think you may be getting my point about the internet. The point is that the internet *is a monopoly*, and it was poorly designed and built and now has become a utility that should be regulated. I say regulated because it has become a tool for Big Tech operators and nothing but a money pit for every consumer accessing it. Our personal monetary values need to grow and cannot maintain that gouging.

This book has twenty-one chapters. I have enjoyed writing eighteen of the twenty-one chapters. This chapter was my least favorite to write about because I *had* to write about this subject matter. The internet has us so entangled in our everyday lives and intersects with almost everything we do or even think about. For many of us using social media for corresponding with friends, or researching subjects, or buying things, the internet works. However, it comes with consequences, mainly expenses. Television for entertainment purposes or getting the latest local and world news also has benefits. Again, there are consequences with them too. I use both venues, the internet and TV, and have been entertained and educated by both. However, it is vitally important we understand the large groups and corporations that are in control of these markets. They naturally want your money, but more importantly they want *as much information about you* as they can get. That information is power for them. It is not just a problem for America, but for the world as well. People have an infatuation with—actually habitual use of—the internet, either with computers or smartphones and large-screen televisions. No pun intended, but we are caught in their web. The personal electronic devices we have been buying, from a consumer's perspective, were designed to help or entertain the consumer—us!—whether the purchase was for personal use or business use. Computers were meant for us to be more productive. In the end, the internet has been a much greater benefit for the manufacturers and not us.

Unfortunately, the tables have turned on us. Being that these devices are electronic, they also are being used to produce data or information about us. We have become so naïve about all the data being produced. A mentor of mine once told me, "Information is power!" What was once a "personal" computer or a television has become a data machine about you for them. Telemarketers, advertising agencies, phone and computer manufacturers want this data about you, because for them it continually enhances any artificial intelligence for their further manipulation of YOU. The limited app and QR code (quick response) pushers know more about your habits than you do. They all have placed us, the consumers or audience, in a position as lab mice or guinea pigs for research, experimentation, and more power. Maybe worse than that, they have access to your money or credit (money that you don't even have yet!). Thank God I did not mention anything about voting machines tied to the internet. Giving the information about us, our habits, etc., to the *wrong people* for the wrong reasons indicates dangerous consequences. These seemingly innocent actions may be used by our nation's adversaries, which they can access, to take down our democracy. Why would these *wrong people* want to do that you might ask? Simply because people like me might suggest that it be strictly regulated because of its flaws and costs. It seems like there is no better way to gain power then to solicit it from your customers as data. What is done with this power (or data) is up to the owners for their discretionary or discriminating purpose, because they most always ask you for your permission to use it. If you don't give your permission do you get the information you need? Sometimes yes and sometimes no. Sounds like cookie practices. Unfortunately, that practice of engaging has a far-reaching exploitation of their audience's thoughts, decisions, and actions. The acts of influencing us by Big Tech and their media business partners was one important motivation to write this book. Like your right to remain silent as Americans when being arrested for crimes, everyone should have their right to have their information from their free thoughts kept silent, not disclosed and NOT USED AGAINST THEM.

When many major TV and cable networks, social media internet outlets, and periodicals began to generate constant negative comments about the sitting elected US President, *it was a clear statement of who controls the media today*. Strong words like *racism* and *fascism* were frequently used by these communication outlets about the US President *before* and *after* his election. These accusations were and remain unfounded. They were formed on bias, trying to create a negative persona. If the media can control your thoughts, they can control your country, and I believe by observation, this is not just a dangerous experiment, but catastrophic. Since 2016, many TV channels and other media have been continually bombarding their audiences with made-up stories. It is amazing what these media giants will do to their viewers. They interpret the events rather than providing information. I learned a long time ago that, "he who pays the piper calls the tune." These many networks and other media should not be telling their employees, the journalists, and especially the front-line reporters what to say. One has to question who is paying the big money to the media outlets for these "staged" scenes instead of providing verifiable facts. I just hope and pray that it is not us, the taxpayers, doling out funding to these mega media giants. That would be adding insult to injury.

From a scientific view, my eyes see how many of today's media are constantly manipulating viewers' thoughts by using psychology, specifically conditioned emotional response, to control listeners' perceptions of events rather than reality, truths, or facts. The question is, are they getting pushed by artificial intelligence for their actions to have a certain outcome develop rather than letting nature take its course? Sounds like another example of self-fulfilling prophecy I discussed in chapter 4 on selfishness.

A century ago, professional journalists would strive for truth before reporting on any news. One may ask, why has reporting the news changed? Why are they attempting to manipulate us today? I can only imagine it is for product or identity marketing, greater power and control in tele-communications, and basically MONEY. Today we are couch potatoes, lab mice, guinea pigs, and have been basically treated as chemicals in test tubes to get the control that these elitists have over us. This lust for control by them is what George Orwell (*1984*) and Aldous Huxley (*Brave New World*) either forewarned or foretold us about in their twentieth-century books. It appears that Big Brother or Big Sister is here in a BIG way. Once you buy into their trap you can't buy your way out, because you do not have enough power, authority, and most importantly leverage (money) to play that game with them. That is because they are taking as much money, specifically your earnings through monthly user fees, your financial security blanket, away from you. You, once referred to as "the customer is king," do not have as much power as they do over you.

In the Soviet Union it was called *Pravda*, their propaganda mega newspaper. Communist Russia used it to control their citizens' thoughts with whatever they wanted to tell them or hide from them—anything that would not be in the government's best interests or objectives. Here in our country, we are talking about some big money by important people who have invested in this media experiment of theirs to control you and profit or benefit by it.

It is sad to think wealthy social ideologists can make their way into our media and have them constantly work to sway public opinion. In case you hear the word *public*, please do not think that it is an abstract thing. I will remind you that you are the public. My Marketing 101 class taught me that you are the target market. I know you are watching TV programs, reading online commercials and thinking you are not really taking in any of that advertising. You also are thinking that the constant pictures and performances being aired by advertisers and their programming contractors are not getting to you. For example, I mentioned in my preface that I see a dichotomy of two centuries, the twentieth and the twenty-first. In the twentieth century, the TV commercials would sell the product. I can recall one aspirin commercial where they showed a cartoon picture of a cross-section of a person's head looking like an anvil, representing the human brain. Then they show a hammer hitting it. Its purpose was to simulate headaches or pain. This advertisement would then suggest to the TV audience to take their pills, and their headaches would go away.

Today, that same aspirin commercial would purposely show a mix of identity groups of people (genders and colors) with headaches sitting around a campfire roasting marshmallows. Then it would show a picture of their product, and somehow everyone is smiling and laughing, jumping up and down, and their headaches are gone. (Maybe it was the marshmallows?) Cecil B. DeMille did not use that many cast members in the movie *Cleopatra*. Twenty years ago, TV commercials typically had one person, known as a "spokesperson." This one person was a well-known, very recognizable and credible person who was used to advertise the products. This type of advertising *worked* and was profitable for the manufacturers. Incidentally, most manufacturers paid for all of the costs and didn't receive any funding from our government for them.

Today, the advertising agencies (and it may only be one for all I know) and networks are selling the great social feeling of *diversity* over the *product*, and are pandering to a TV audience about their product making them feel socially good instead of what their product does. I have observed these commercials countless times over the past ten years, and I know the scientific field's use of conditioned emotional response. I discussed that in chapter 1. It is so blatant that I do not even need a data collection sheet to record this data. If I tried, I would never have had time to write this book. As a potential customer for a product or service I do not need a mob of people to sell it to me. The manufacturer, their distribution network, and most importantly the potential consumer wants to know what the product will do for them… period. It appears that it is more important to get a social messages out by the types of groups cast in the commercials then it is to sell the advertised products. What is really the target market in TV advertising? Is it for the entertainment for special interest groups or the manufactured products' intended purpose which may be needs based for their customers? Are the advertised products the secondary point in these commercials? Whatever happened to the customer "being king" in the field of sales philosophy? I know for a fact that the advertisers are getting federal money for placing "diversity" in their advertisements. The tables have turned when the advertisers *and the government* are the "kings" over the potential customer. The biggest insult is when the advertisers' and networks' customers, the products' manufacturers, themselves get shafted (beer lite).

The subject above was only about TV commercials. I did not even mention all the advertisements being done on the internet. Most marketing firms using the internet know they have reached the nirvana heights of internet marketing exposure. That is because of their top status on the search engine listings; it ensures their "hits" get continually higher and makes other business's attempts at competition almost impossible. Therefore, the internet and those large money-making firms are "all in" with keeping the status quo and keeping out any newbies. The lack of marketing access is a big problem with its design flaw and expense for its users. Another flaw: the power of algorithms allows for poorly made products that you buy from pictures on small LCD screens instead of three-dimensional ones in stores. The devices we once called our cell phones have really turned into sell phones. I discuss in more detail the problems with internet buying in later chapters.

The TV-watching audience can be influenced by networks and advertisers and many times are only interested in the emotional responses from their programs. The feedback they receive from your responses may actually work to influence you more and more. You need to watch this type of advertising and ask yourself, what are they really selling? Is it the product or social commentary? Surely we can all think and evaluate products ourselves without our government muddying it up. I mentioned before that our government, your tax money, is giving corporations money to advertise "diversity." Advertisers and their media marketers should stop trying to sell some sick mind-controlling form of what they are calling diversity. It is not diverse because it is not truly a cross-sectional demographic and not all-inclusive. This type of diversity is designed to be biased against one segment of our society. By now most Americans have seen this fake diversity at work and seen it at almost all school levels. After these few years of this biased diversity training, we understand their objectives are to prey on one's emotional feelings from a historical point of view. If you ever had this type of "diversity training," you get the point and the presenter's point. Some group is offended, so they think that you do not understand them. Yes, we do understand there are social problems and a lack of understanding between groups. Hell, there is a lack of understanding between people living on the same street or even in the same household. The type of diversity training as presented today only clouds the real issue, and that is *respect*, not just for some cultural claim but for *all people* as individuals.

What you are seeing is what the mechanical Ben said at the American history theme park I mentioned earlier. That is, "America is the great experiment in democracy." Unfortunately for us, the TV and internet users, we are finding that this marketing experiment, in an effort to push many other purposes like politics and diversity, may be causing damage. Whoever owns these advertising firms is probably laughing all the way to the bank though. These misdirected people do not understand the amount of mental cruelty that they may be causing, or they are purposely doing it for some political or cultural gain, and doing it with our tax money! Specifically, it is *the stereotyping of people in the casting of the actors in their roles.* Stereotyping is defined as a standard mental picture held in common by social members of a group and represents an oversimplified opinion, prejudiced attitude, or uncritical judgement. These advertisers almost always cast a person from one social group that gets matched up with a person from a different social group. The first role most often is the genius hero and typically of a minority group color. Another group, typically male, is cast as the clown, comedian, geek/nerd, or weirdo. No need for clown makeup by now; after these few years of witnessing this stereotyping we know all too well who this social group is: the one targeted to be CULTURALLY CANCELLED. Before one word is uttered out of that actor's mouth, the audience knows and expects it to be some stupid, funny, or clown's comment; that or they will have a pie thrown in their face. The advertisers forget that continually casting these groups of people as clowns/nerds/undesirables might just offend that group of people. Actually, continuing to cast that group of people in those roles is an act of discrimination. The Civil Rights Act indicates that these casting acts are acts of group discrimination.

Here is the main problem. The kids and adolescents today see these stereotypes and look to see where they fit in. If they see themselves cast as a clown or stupid, that's the big problem based on one's self-esteem. That demeaning act is a problem and grows into mental and emotional ones. I have observed that many TV commercials typically do not portray black women and lighter men equally to darker men and lighter women. We have to ask ourselves the question, "Are the media influencers casting certain types of people as 'bad seeds'? Are they attempting to have them shunned by others? Hitler and Stalin did this. It was called genocide!

This type of genocide is an electronic mind-game to shun one group of people and make another group think they have an increase in status, power, and perhaps political leverage. Why would the people pushing this type of advertising do this? Perhaps because the political party that supplied the funding for this type of advertising is betting that it can influence groups of their listeners with a way of cancelling out other groups. They know that their political group has traditionally voted for them, and their return on their investment (our tax money) will achieve votes going their way. However, it is only bull-jive, folks. They are only visual scenes on LCD screens. The mostly featured group in these ads has not gained any more power, but inflation that an influencing party created since 2021 has caused less power (money) for that already economically challenged people. Only the elites in Big Tech and the media's partners gain more power, and they still want more. It's right back to the ghetto after all the voting is done! It is the same type of gimmicks that that party has been using for a hundred years over minorities. They act or say they are going to improve welfare for all minorities, but it is only a perception and not the reality. That party does very little except to help themselves and their big-money backers. After one hundred years, American minorities are finally seeing the realities of that party's bull and are now hip to their jive.

A possible fix to TV and internet advertising shenanigans should be a system of randomly cast roles for all people in media advertising. There is too much stereotyping of people, and these are acts of discrimination. Randomly cast roles would show that groups are not being discriminated against. Advertisers may be fanning the flames of racial or gender bias. Why don't they simply return to having product "spokespersons" for their advertising needs and save on the acting labor costs? Or even better, use cartoons instead of live actors for comic relief in their commercials. If the advertisers continually push this fake cultural diversity on their paying customers, my only suggestion is to *boycott* the advertised products if they offend you.

I understand that some advertising agencies get their information about demographics from polling organizations. Questions should be asked of the pollsters as to the details of the populations that are being interviewed for their data. Did you know that one of the largest data service companies is owned by a company in Communist China? That is a scary thought, that foreign companies possibly provide data to advertisers to show what should be painted across our large TV screens or small smartphones.

Real diversity respects all humans and does not look to ostracize people for their differences. As the songwriter Ray Stevens wrote, everything (everyone) is beautiful in its (their) own way. Just sell the products and no more social-group stereotyping, please!

Since the cable networks believe they have total control over advertising to use it for racial discrimination purposes, I propose that a new type of TV broadcasting be developed without advertising. It would be a pay-it-forward system by consumers for having no advertising. It would be similar to the commercial-free radio we now enjoy. It would be serious TV. It could possibly be done using satellite-dish operations, keeping it separate from cable TV and competitive with satellite TV.

For this chapter, my inspiration to write it came from the songs "Dirty Laundry," sung by Don Henley and written by Don Henley and Danny Kortchmar, and "It's Only Make Believe," sung by Conway Twitty and written by Conway Twitty and Jack Nance. In "Dirty Laundry," the singer tells us it is all about only the sensational stories and keeping TV audiences engaged. Conway Twitty's song reminds me of how much I love America and that there are powerful groups out there that use whatever means—like discrimination, which is illegal and unethical—to make money. Especially when they can use our tax money to help pay for their product's advertising. I hope the readers understand after reading about the affects that our nations media can have on their viewer's psyche they see the importance between observations and discrimination.

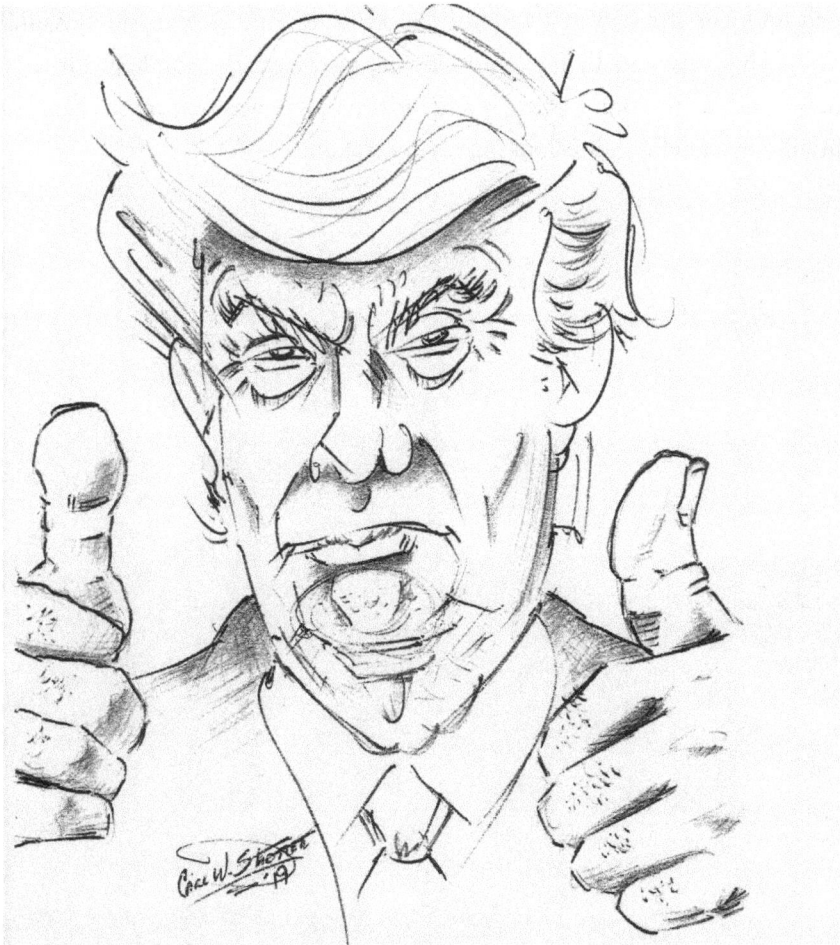

I was born in Cleveland, Ohio. I am proud of that heritage. Ohio politically has been a bellwether state when predicting US presidential elections. In fact, since the 1960 presidential election, Ohio has had a streak of accurate predictions, except for the 2020 election of Joe Biden. I am not sure if Donald Trump will even be able to run again for US president. If not, he probably will go down in our history as being the greatest living political martyr. I believe his voters knew in 2016 it was about a better plan, and not the man. In a 1960s film starting actress Haley Mills as a Pollyanna, she said that Abraham Lincoln had a saying. It was "When you look for the bad in mankind expecting to find it, you surely will." The saying was actually fabricated for the movie script. Abraham Lincoln never said it. The point being made for the movie was that none of us are infallible; therefore, quit looking for those failures.

# 6.

# Distractions to Your Goals

I loved my mother dearly, and I could not think of a more family-oriented, selfless person, other than perhaps my wife. My wife often tells me that I am so negative. It is not that I am so negative, it is that she is so positive. She has such a great attitude and has been a great inspiration for me. However, I believe everyone has vices, and I do believe people need and deserve a break. My mom's distraction was the daily newspaper. As a child, when I needed her attention to resolve an important issue, my mom would be concentrating on some newspaper article—at least it seemed that way when I wanted her attention. She probably was looking at the grocery store ads, trying to save a couple of pennies from food coupons, or what were called green stamps, so our family could make ends meet. Family debt wasn't an option, *it wasn't even thought of* because of the uncertainties of paying it off.

Today, with the advent smartphones, we are getting blinked, buzzed, ringed, honked at, or whatever about what God only knows may be some life-threatening information. Habitually we immediately stop and peek at it, or our world will end. Hell, we cannot even continue driving our cars without looking at these distractions... LOOK OUT!

Our smart phone is an example of one of the biggest problems we have today. Lord, please free us from these pocket-sized LCD screen distractions so we can focus on the issues that we have planned for in our BIG picture for ourselves. Do not let social media, the motion picture industry, TV, magazines, newspapers, and especially advertising affect your goals.

Those media industries just might be against a person with your looks or beliefs and lure you into hate or question your societal values. It is a trick to sway you… but stay focused and stay the course. One of my favorite actors who portrayed Nelson Mandela in a presentation of him said, and I paraphrase, that you are the master of your own fate and the captain of your soul. Meaning that as long as we have the *freedom* to do it, we can have our rights to life, liberty, and the pursuit to happiness. Remember, as far as the media is concerned, you are just a marketing tool, and no more than a lab rat for their ratings or the manipulating of consumers.

So here we are today, tied at the hip with these new technologies we have. Unfortunately, technology has created more problems for us instead of solutions. We must learn to use these technologies *to our advantage* and not be a *slave to them* but rather their masters.

If you are a social media junkie, start your goals by mostly going to career articles. Pay attention to how much time you are wasting surfing "stuff" to increase your debt. Smartphones usually have calendars and can also tell you how much time you have been spending on them. List all your important tasks and activities on the calendars and have reminders come to aid you. Take the time, sort out those activities and prioritize them, and do NOT—I repeat, do NOT—list things that could be a distraction to you and limit your constructive goals. Stop going to the casino, drinking alcohol, or using vaping products. These items should not be listed on your organizing calendars. Hell, *they are not supposed to be on your mind*. If they are, you need to add something especially important on your calendar: an appointment with a trained professional to help you. That was not a joke. I am serious! *You are hooked*. You cannot let go. You have an addiction to whatever is consuming your thoughts, and more importantly your time. These things will point you downward quicker than a divining rod over a water main (you probably will have to research "divining rod"). Your habit is not just some fashionable thing. We will discuss in our next chapter on the latest statistics about the deadly abusive quantities of drugs and alcohol taken and their adverse effect on the people of our beautiful country.

Before you move toward your new goals, it is wise to take a hard look at where you are now. I do not want to scare you like the ghost of Christmas future. It did scare Ebenezer Scrooge in *A Christmas Carol,* but this is especially important for you. Look at your friends. Are they really your friends or are they your frenemies? People like that are only boat anchors tied around you. They could be pulling you down only to raise their own status. What about your parents? Do they really care? If you just turned eighteen, are they only glad at not having to pay alimony from their divorce decree? Who are your real mentors? Maybe it is or was your grandparents. They most probably came from a generation that really cared for something other than themselves.

Are you drinking and doing drugs? Are you gaming too much? Just because the corner gas station has lottery tickets, cigarettes, vaping products, and booze does not mean it is an acceptable habit. It just means that the gas station owner wants to make money. If you want to get somewhere in your life, leave those habits behind. Those habits will take your new goals in the wrong direction. You have to get straight because your own weaknesses are dragging you down. Statistics show that fantasy sports are a waste of time. Making excuses for yourself does not help either. When it seems hopeless, think about joining any branch of the US military. They need you, and the experience and discipline that is inherent there has helped millions of young men and women find fulfilling careers and improve their lives. That has worked especially for minorities. The GI Bill has led many to higher education and even helped them earn a college degree at NO COST!

God did not put you on this earth so you could be unproductive or a burden on others. You are God's gift. You are a thinking, breathing, loving creation. God created you in his own image, and he was a creator; therefore, so are you. YOU, my friend, are as Dr. Frankenstein so scientifically put it when he created his monster: "ALIVE!" God did not create you to be the next victim on some evil zealot's death list, or the television or internet's targeted marketing piece of data. You should be a productive, self-actuating being. What is your vocational goal? If you say a doctor or lawyer, you might want to rethink your goals. These two careers are high paying and popular, but expensive. There are many others who initially chose that path and found themselves without a degree and with a mountain of college debt. Find a career that would be meaningful to you. Consider the arts or education. There are plenty of career opportunities. Start out in a small job that may be closely related to your goal(s). You may not realize it, but that job could be a springboard to an unexpected interest for you, one that you may have never realized.

One of my daughters started her career that way. While in college, she wanted to be a teacher. While attending college she worked part-time at a restaurant to make some extra spending money. After graduation she took a job as a bank teller. An opportunity came up to be a flight attendant at a major airline's smaller division. With her background in food service, combined with her money-handling experience, she was in a good position to "land" the job, and she did! Now she is flying the friendly skies and whistling while she works.

Start your career adventure by networking. You probably have access to a computer. If not, get a library card from your local library. Use their computers to get on your way. Contact companies, schools, or professional associations about their job opportunities or how to get into the business. There are plenty of people to help you.

I recommend that you schedule an appointment with your high school guidance counselor. With the school lockdowns today, it may be an after-school appointment. Start out by asking how things are progressing at the school. Explain your thoughts about a career and ask for suggestions. Be sure to provide enough information as to how and where a prospective employer can contact you. Start contacting organizations about careers that interest you.

If you have been recently laid off or unemployed, do not hesitate to contact your state for their procedures to claim unemployment compensation. Not all states have the same procedures and requirements. Read your state's requirements carefully. In some states, time is of the essence to register.

Many people of retirement age who have left the job market can, if they choose, find gratifying employment. I know from firsthand experience that you may not be ready for full-time retirement. You may have underestimated your retirement income, or want more conveniences during your retirement, or have an unforeseen expense. There are many online employment agencies out there that solicit local businesses in your area for part-time employees or, if you choose, a full-time position.

Some questions or concerns people should consider before seeking employment are: 1) Do you have the stamina for the desired position? 2) Does re-employment adversely affect any present retirement benefits? Some states have penalties for reemployment. 3) Are you familiar enough with the type of work that it will not cause you mental stress? 4) How do family members feel about your decision about reemployment? 5) Will you needing to purchase a car and pay for its insurance and maintenance? Is public transit an option? Having to work for extra money can be as much of a problem as a solution.

I hope this chapter has reenergized your life's goals. Life is God's gift to our world, and we must be the gatekeepers to maintain its wonders. As the rock group Jefferson Airplane said in the title song from one of their albums, "You Are the Crown of Creation." My mother-in-law has a saying: "Idle hands are the devil's workshop!" Although a common saying many years ago, it has a practical social meaning. If you are not keeping busy, for whatever reason, there is a likelihood for negative thoughts about your inactivity or your life's path. Therefore, keep physically busy and avoid any electronic-tool activities, and this will eliminate the possibility for any negativity.

Being an observer of this wonderful world is a pleasurable act; however, it is everyone's responsibility to sustain it. It is like we said in chapter 3, discussing the musical *The Sound of Music*: Nothing comes from nothing and never will. Take a tip from me and others and find employment where you can be happy so you can whistle while you work!

For this chapter, my inspiration came from the songs "I Can See for Miles" and "I Can See Clearly Now." "I Can See for Miles" was written by Peter Townshend and performed by the Who. They sing that the Eiffel Tower and the Taj Mahal can be seen on clear days. Large objects and wonders of the world like that can be in your personal goals, but only if you try. I believe it was Walt Disney who said if you can dream it you can do it. If you get yourself straight you will not need a crystal ball to see your goals more clearly. "I Can See Clearly Now" was written and sung by Johnny Nash. He says if you look straight ahead there will be nothing but blue skies for you. It can be all blue skies if you do look straight ahead and keep on pushing toward your career goals and finally achieve them. *They are straight ahead.*

# 7.

# Our Drugged Society

In chapter 1 of this book we referenced observations and the scientific method, English logic, and making decisions based on information. In this chapter we will focus on those principals by emphasizing important data about America today.

Everyone is talking about the opioid epidemic, and rightly so. It is not only killing its victims, but causing unbelievable collateral damage to families, friends, and our environment. The death rate from opioids and other drug abuse has risen from almost 20,000 in the year 2000, to over 70,000 in 2019, and a whopping 102,000 in 2021. That is over five times the number of deaths since 2000. It is not just about the deaths. The drugs that we are taking end up in our water supply. This topic will be discussed in the chapter on our environment.

I am a find-the-root-cause person and would like to begin with some reasons for our drug problems today. Let me identify each of the drug problems and look at possible theories to help correct them. One fact that I know, based on data over the last twenty years, is that we have an abuse of recreational stimulants today. Our first stimulant observation is the legally obtained and supposedly innocent drug, alcohol.

[1]The definition for *stimulant*, from a dictionary, is an agent (such as a drug) that produces a temporary increase of the functional activity or efficiency of an organism or any of its parts. For example, an alcoholic beverage.

History has told us that mankind has consumed alcohol through eating fermented fruit for thousands of years. Many ancient cultures have used variations of fruits, wheat, and barley to make and drink alcohol. So much for the history of alcohol. Scientists will tell you that there are latent cancer cells in all of us, and when activated... look out! That is how the addiction to alcohol is. Once you become addicted to it, your life and the lives of others around you become adversely affected.

Most people do not know their own metabolic tolerance or physical limitations to drinking alcohol. The amount of alcohol consumed affects each of us differently because of different factors. However, recovering from its effect is pretty much consistent with how much sleep we get after consuming it. Some recent governmental statistics on alcohol tell us this:

- Alcohol-impaired driving accounts for 30 percent of all driving fatalities each year.
- More than 15 million people struggle with an alcohol use disorder in the US, but less than 8 percent of those receive treatment.
- Recently more than 65 million Americans report binge drinking, which is more than 40 percent of the total of current alcohol users.
- Teen alcohol use kills 4,700 teens each year.
- Drunk driving costs the US more than $199 billion every year.
- Alcohol abuse disorder in women has increased by 83.7 percent between 2002 and 2013 according to a study back then.
- High-risk drinking, defined as more than three drinks in a day or seven in a week for women, is on the rise among women, by about 58 percent, according to a 2017 study comparing habits from 2001 and 2013.
- More than 45 percent of adult women report drinking alcohol recently, and 12 percent of these report binge drinking.
- Binge drinking dramatically increases the risk of sexual assaults on women, *especially those living in a college campus setting.*

- Women who binge drink are more likely to have *unprotected sex, increasing the risk of unintended pregnancy and sexually transmitted diseases.* It can interrupt the menstrual cycle and lead to infertility.
- Approximately one in two women of childbearing age drink, and 18 percent of women binge drink. For pregnant women this can increase the risk of fetal alcohol syndrome, which can cause mental and physical birth defects.

It seems to me that as parents we are all too quick to see our children grow up and be "somebody." Many of us leave our children's guidance to childcare workers for most of their day (except when they sleep). This cycle for most Americans is from cradle to high school graduation. You can be an inspiration to your children while they are young and guide them away from the pitfalls of alcohol abuse. They need direction on the right decisions for them to make regarding the drinking of alcohol. Decision-making does not come from osmosis. Shipping them off to some faraway college after their high school graduation without a clear significant message about the dangers of drug and alcohol abuse only compounds our society's problems in these areas. Options for the immature high school graduates can be for non-college-degree careers closer to home. Statistically speaking, due to the ever-increasing amount of drug and alcohol abuse in our nation, that option may just keep your adult children healthier, safer, and economically debt-free until they mature more.

I really care about our families and friends, and I really care about our nation's health specifically. There is a time for work and a time for play. The question is how much your play or recreation effects your work. Hell, how much does your play affect your life?

Did you know that the sale of alcoholic beverages has doubled since 2002? Doubled. That is alarming because it is not like we just came out of an alcohol prohibition in 2002, as our nation did in 1933. Since the

1850s the alcohol consumption rate per capita had pretty much remained the same until 1933, and then leveled off again to until 2002.

Today, alcoholism is also known as alcohol use disorder. It is a broad term for any drinking of alcohol that results in mental or physical health problems. The disorder is divided into two types: alcohol abuse and alcohol dependence. In a medical context, alcoholism is said to exist when two or more of the following conditions are present. A person drinks large amounts of alcohol over a long period of time and has difficulty stopping. An alcoholic spends an enormous amount of time purchasing and consuming alcohol and fails to fulfill responsibilities, especially their own healthcare.

Alcohol usage results in social problems, health problems, and risky situations. Withdrawal occurs when people stop consuming it, because alcohol tolerance reoccurs with its use.

What is causing this craving for stimulants today? The answer is YOU. It is a typical cause-effect situation. It is our free society. It is your choice. It is your body. It is your mind, and *you* are "out of control," right? Wrong. When your selfish behavior is out of control and starts to affect your job, your family, and everyone around you, measures must be taken, boys and girls. Your alcohol problem can affect other people and their control of their own behavior. You may be depressed. Your job and/or family situation and listening to the made-up news on various media today can be depressing. COVID-19 has caused unemployment and disrupted social contact and many of our normal routines and behaviors. Many are still feeling the effects from the pandemic. There may even be some hooked on alcohol because they are not having any drug or alcohol testing done to them, *especially from those working remotely*. Out of sight, out of mind. That's a great new American management philosophy. Discovering that someone has a problem is the first step to recovery. Employers should be aware that some of their working-from-home employees may be hiding their dependence on alcohol.

If you suspect that you are dependent on alcohol or drugs, see a doctor about it. However, do not expect them to prescribe a pill for this problem. Why? That would be like adding insult to injury. Whatever you do, do not mix alcohol with drugs. These mixtures cause physical and mental issues. Your head and your liver will be negatively affected. If you know someone with recent serious behavior issues and you suspect it is caused by drug or alcohol abuse, suggest that they seek help. Explain that they should tell their doctor about their recent behavior changes. Hopefully, their doctor will recommend further treatment. You should try to help people enjoy life's pleasures without the impairments that alcohol and drug abuse can cause.

The need for America to have recreational marijuana and legalized drugs for the freedom to increase our suicide rate has me scratching my head. It started me thinking that there are basically two groups of people. One is the group that cares about people—their mental, physical, and spiritual being. The second group of people only think about themselves, they are the rich and powerful, and have zero regard for the ill effects they may cause to our society. The biggest benefit to legalizing marijuana is for the powerful and rich. People are hooked on drugs and alcohol because they become *impaired*. That particular group of rich and powerful people are no better than drug pushers. These selfish acts relate to legalized gambling as well. When I was growing up in the '60s and '70s, there were only two states that had legalized gambling, Nevada and New Jersey. I guess their border states became envious of the amount of increased tax revenue and business boom that their neighboring states were benefiting from, so they legalized it too. My state of Ohio only made gambling legal because Pennsylvania, Indiana, and Michigan already had it.

Legalizing marijuana in each state is the same deal. The dope is being grown, and the growers have BIG money backing. Those growers are lobbying state legislators on how much states like Colorado are making on it. Now, this is just innocent lobbying of course—no dinners, no quid pro quo, etc. It is unfortunate that our society is bending on our children's mental health and even considering taking our states to a new "high." Many parents have problems with their kids getting drunk on alcohol, now they must worry about them getting even higher. What is next? Legalizing cocaine and prostitution? Why not? It could be a real big money maker for the states. I believe one presidential candidate proposed legalizing prostitution during the 2020 election race. These actions are destructive progressivism. That is not progress…it is regress. We must start being vigilant in identifying when businesses collude with politicians in their states and in our federal government to legalize any form of drugs, whether they be opioids, marijuana, or vaping products. They call it lobbying. That is just another dangerous *soft and fuzzy* word in the destructive progressivism vocabulary. Many of these drug products are taken into the lungs, and during these variant virus health concerns, having clean, healthy lungs can be a lifesaver.

I cannot for the life of me understand how these states like California and Colorado could legalize the smoking of marijuana and call it a *recreational* drug. I coached recreational baseball and softball for twenty-five years and have a whole different understanding of what *recreational* means. The lobbyists and the liberals sure like using those *soft* words today. Unfortunately, it is those soft words that are usually lethal. They are words created by smooth politicians and salesmen, again, as stated in these cases, they are nothing but **drug pushers**. When it comes to legalizing the ingestion of tetrahydrocannabinol, or THC, it is not a healthy choice. THC is the chemical component in marijuana. I am totally against legalizing any form of THC as it relates to *ingesting* it into your body (or mind). If you want to use it as a salve for your sore knees or joints, I am fine with that. Do not put it *into* your body as a stimulant to alter your senses. We have enough problems in America through this post-COVID period when it comes to mental illness and stress. I guess states like Colorado want to be as socially cool as California. As for treating mental health there are proven effective drugs other than THC to combat this growing problem.

We know for a fact that too many people get behind the wheel of a car when they are over the legal blood alcohol limits. You must be careful when choosing who you socialize with. Many times when groups of young adults combine socializing with alcohol and drugs it can lead to big trouble. It may even lead to drug abuse over something as simple as a dare. The fact is, when socializing with your friends, folks pretty much are "into" the same things. The young and vulnerable want to appear to be more mature. *However, they are at an experimental age.* That is a key point. The difference between *acting* mature and *being* mature is to know yourself. Once you know yourself, your strengths and weaknesses, then you will know how to make the right decisions in life. That is being mature, and keeping with that trend makes you wise.

My inspiration for writing this chapter came from the songs "I Want To Take You Higher" and "Kicks." "I Want To Take You Higher" was written by Sylvester Stewart and performed by Sly and the Family Stone. They sing about wanting to get higher and higher. Why do people do this? The reasons are that their tolerance levels to drugs and alcohol become altered after many uses of either or both. Some people need increased amounts of a drug or drugs to return to the height of the "high." The height is their state of comfort, or could even be the euphoria or nirvana they mentally wish to return to. If they cannot return to it with the same amount of drugs or alcohol consumed, they resort to taking more and more until it is achieved. That is when their body and/or mind reaches a dangerous "critical mass." That is when it becomes either a health crisis or even death.

The song "Kicks," written by Barry Mann and Cynthia Weil and performed by Paul Revere and the Raiders, influenced me because it tells about using drugs or alcohol as the accelerants to "kick in" the feeling of paradise. However, that feeling only lasts so long. The song describes the next day after your high when you wake up feeling worse than the day before. This becomes a continuing cycle for drug abusers. It continues because drug abusers are impaired and can't objectively see clearly that they are hooked. The addicted keep attempting to reach their paradise, which unfortunately is only temporary, is less and less reachable, and can cause death.

# 8.

# When Cool Is Not Cool

I once made a very sarcastic remark about having our American flag display the President of the United States smoking a joint of marijuana on the back of Old Glory's field of red, white, and blue. How cool is that? Of course it was all meant in jest. However, with Colorado, California, and others lining their states' coffers with all that tax money they are collecting from dope sales, the "Cool Flag" seems appropriate. I wonder when all their neighboring states will catch on to this golden goose moneymaker. I cannot wait for the advertising commercials for these sales. They'll probably have a carnival barker that spouts, "Hurry, hurry, step right up. Welcome to our big top. While inside you can see our three-ring circus of spaced-out clowns, watch Alice smoking a hookah pipe, and enjoy an interactive giant bar complete with go-go dancers for each patron." Is that us? What is with the hurry to be cool? What is the hurry to become a third-world nation? This is when *cool is not cool*.

It is sad to know that a worldwide epidemic had to happen for people to grasp the importance of good health. It was gratifying to see Surgeon General Dr. Jerome Adams discuss the importance of practicing rational measures to insure everyone's health through the COVID-19 pandemic. He told our communities basically that we must change the way we socialize to stop the spread of COVID-19. He suggested no large gatherings and limiting alcohol and other intoxicants. Why? All Americans with their many backgrounds must be strong and healthy to fight off not just the COVID virus but all potential diseases and viruses.

These healthy changes may not be cool, but they are smart. That is the point of this chapter.

Today, being cool can get you killed. If it does not kill you, it can kill your parents, grandparents, friends, or coworkers. It's about time we all start thinking more about being smarter and less about being cooler. *Cool is for the kids that do not know any better. Cool* is the word used when someone cannot articulate the correct description of someone or something. Being smart is what Americans are all about, right? We all need to better ourselves and get a broader education. Why did Dr. Martin Luther King preach? Why did Anna Maxwell lead the way in nursing? Why did Charles Lindbergh fly across the Atlantic Ocean? What about our race to space? Is this who we are—a bunch of dopeheads? You let yourself and your country down by legalizing harmful "recreational" drugs. We must remember that THC when ingested is a psychoactive drug.

The states that are legalizing dope do not care about their people holistically. These legislators—and believe me, they are exceptionally good salespeople—are more interested in using your hard-earned money to increase your taxes for their pet projects. Of course, increasing the size of government for them to play *with your money* will include a well-earned pay raise for themselves. These types of elected officials are the self-servicing variety. Your health is way down on their list. God bless the elected officials that are doing their job in representing you and your vision for our country. I am sure you want to get your money's worth out of them representing you. We will discuss the subjects of government and health in later chapters.

Adolescents are so susceptible to peer pressure. It happens to most youngsters. Parents that teach their children about the importance of family over friends have the right solutions. These children usually stay out of big trouble. My father would often tell me that having friends is not that important in life. I was fortunate to have both: a strong family bond and good friends. I am not saying I did not get into trouble; I did and so did my friends. If you think you were cool, my friends and I thought we were the coolest. We jokingly called ourselves the Parrello Brothers. We had the cars, we had the girlfriends, and we had a lot of laughs too. Those kinds of friendships last a lifetime, and so do the memories. However, it is important to know the right things to do, and hopefully all our children will eventually mature into good solid citizens.

Later in my life, my wife and I had four children, and in 1987 I was introduced to Cub Scouting. My two boys each joined the Cub Scouts and later became Boy Scouts. I even became a Scoutmaster for a few years. As a Scoutmaster, parents would ask me if the Boy Scouts was a *cool* experience for their boys. I would always tell them, "Scouting is *fun*, not cool." Scouting for children was and still is fun. I had two daughters in Girl Scouts, and my wife was a troop leader. In fact, my oldest daughter is a Girl Scout troop leader, and my oldest son is a scout leader in my grandsons' scouting programs. The scouting activities children and young adults learn are challenging activities and important lifelong skills—in some cases lifesaving skills. The most important lesson learned is the camaraderie that the group shares with each other. Children can still have a lot of fun today without being cool.

What is with this "cool" thing anyway? [1]A dictionary defines the word cool as: 1. a state moderately cold and lacking in warmth. 2. acting dispassionate, having calmness and self-control. 3. Cool can also mean lacking friendliness. 4. In music, like jazz, *cool* means having restrained emotion and frequent use of counterpoint. However, the meaning probably most used today is to be fashionable or popular. I suppose any one of these descriptions for *cool* just makes you want to join the cool club.

I know we have fifty states, and it's only a few of them, but the money grabbing legislators that think they know what is best for you *and your children* will go to their grave telling you that these money-making wonder drugs will generate so much revenue for your state that it will be listed in *Fortune* magazine's Global 500 list. Your state will be so rich, you will not have to work anymore. Wow, how cool is that? My wife always says to me, "Alan, if sounds too good to be true, it probably is." You know, she is always right about that. When the politicians get up on their soapboxes and start their election campaigns, everyone should listen to my wife. So, scouts and non-scouts, be prepared (the scout motto). Listen to the *critical issues* that affect you, your family, your employment/career, your taxes, and your healthcare costs. One's livelihood is the important piece of the puzzle that can give you peace of mind. Intangible things like the Green New Deal, without knowing all the facts, is an example. These issues should be way down on your list. As far as global warming goes, you cannot predict sunspots, and one theory says that sunspots may have caused the Ice Age. Every American should be cognizant of *pollution* first before a Green New Deal, which is supposedly about climate change. Americans are not being told about how the costs will ultimately take our nation down. Where are the details for this "cool" program? We haven't been given all the details of it. It almost sounds like "taxation without *presentation*." We need to begin the mitigation of pollution at every state level first. We need to use any money earmarked for climate change, or whatever they call the overpriced act to reengineer our large cities, and design them for better public transit and interstate rail transportation, then make them safer, healthier, and better places to live and work in. I discuss pollution and our environment in detail in chapter 18.

There have been many controversial studies about marijuana not being a gateway drug. The latest studies show that marijuana, alcohol, and nicotine are *all* gateways to harder drugs like opioids and cocaine. I do not think young people today are familiar with the many movies made about drug abuse. One of my favorites is Frank Sinatra in *The Man with the Golden Arm*. He plays the part of a 1950s musician hooked on drugs, which are keeping him from his potentially great musical career.

Another movie titled *Flowers of Darkness* is a documentary narrated by Paul Newman. Paul lost his only son to a drug overdose. In this 1972 documentary Paul discusses where opium is grown, made into heroin, shipped, and distributed. The movie told about opium's addicting effects on Americans. That was in 1972. For your information, the largest growers of opium were in...*Afghanistan*! I will try not to make any connections to why we were so eager to run from there. Do you think the World Health Organization should fix the monumental drug issues of our world? That would be a noble goal of theirs for sure.

We all know too well the devastating effects opioids have had on America these past twenty years. The increase of social media's influence on family members *may* also be a contributing factor to the increase in drug and alcohol use (social pressure). What about your family's peer groups picking on them and saying they are not "cool" enough? OMG! We must grow up and be smarter and work harder. Can't we have fun without being "cool"?

Most of the children's programs today aired on television are prioritizing social interaction of special interest groups over family. You very rarely see a family scene on television programming. Why not emphasize strong family values? These Hollywood productions, or even the ones produced in New York, do not do this anymore. To the unsuspecting adult viewer it is just another kid program. The technical problem with this attempt though is what I call "mis-diversity." I am again mentioning the TV commercials discussed in chapter 5 about social media. A discrimination problem exists with the way various special interest groups are cast. There is a definite stereotyping of the cast members, whether they are the children performing in studio programming or even the cartoons. The hero roles always seem to go to one type of group, and the clown/nerd roles always seem to go to another identifiable group. Unfortunately, the viewing children see themselves fitting or not fitting in these various roles, and that is the problem. This mis-diversity attempts to ostracize one particular set of cast members. Programs that ostracize, especially children, can be mentally damaging to the viewing audience, not to mention the cast players. Being ostracized *is the gateway* to mental health issues and social hate. The cool identity groups of today that push "cancel culture" are the biggest cultivators of ostracism and *may be* attempting to create or cultivate hate among the ostracized.

I know what you are thinking. "Hey, this guy says he practices being scientific. How is he measuring the amount of coolness from these kid TV shows?" That is simple. I am a licensed parent and responsible for my children's input, much like you track your computer's input. You know—garbage in, garbage out. All the TV shows are trying to push is a group-socializing thing. I know the TV sitcoms *Friends* and *Seinfeld* were very popular, but they were for adult entertainment. Our easily influenced kids are watching TV programs based on the lifestyles of the large markets in New York City and Los Angeles. In between those two large-market centers there is a vast area called the rest of the United States. Okay, so the TV shows *Lassie, Rin Tin Tin,* and *The Littlest Hobo* (about a stray German shepherd) may not be the coolest shows for children. However, TV shows about nature, animals, and people in real environmental settings, away from studio-produced shows, are entertaining for kids and a break from the "come join my cool friends" push.

I believe, and I hope you also believe, that kids today need better role models. When you think about it, we adults are no different than our children. Everybody is trying to be cool. *It is so fashionable now.* It is *in*, it is *now*, and it is *wild.* I love that word *fashionable.* It reminds me of my first job I had in the public sector. A bunch of us workers snuck off to the local snack shop around the corner from where we were working in East Cleveland. The supervisor brought me into his office and asked where I had gone. I told him, "I was following the rest of the sheep, and went to the snack shop." He gave me a warning and said, "Look, you are new here. I am telling you now, keep it up and you'll be following the sheep to slaughter."

It is an interesting oxymoron about the credo of the "cool" people. They expect everything in life to be *accepted by everyone.* However, for some reason these same people absolutely cannot accept the fact that many people do not believe in accepting everything. As a consumer and taxpayer, I cannot and will never accept bad customer service, either from large corporations, their foreign partnerships, or any of our local, state, or federal governments. We pay high amounts of our wages in taxes, and we should expect quality workmanship and performance. Corporations and our governments today seem to purposely agitate many of their customers (taxpayers) with shoddy products and services, especially in their telecommunication services by contracting that important service out to overseas contractors. I honestly believe this is an effort to totally dismantle our telephone services and replace it with artificial intelligence chatbots. AI chatbots DO NOT WORK because they do not "hit" on the exact point we are attempting to explain. In these cases, not getting the specific important feedback on the problem/issue usually causes even more mistakes or shows their customer what they really think of them. Not accepting everything may not be cool, *but it is wise.*

For this chapter, the music that inspired me to write it came from the songs "In the Ghetto" written by Mac Davis and sung by Elvis Presley, and "Straight Ahead" written and performed by Jimi Hendrix. A very important message is taken from "In the Ghetto." That is, we have many major issues in our big cities today that go far beyond the need to drive electric cars. These people in the inner city are suffering—economically, yes, but culturally as well. There is nothing "cool" about suffering. Only positive action and not words or attitudes get things done. Make no mistake: However small, all actions take energy. It is not the time to stifle domestic energy sources. As in the song from chapter 3, "Something Good," we learned that nothing comes from nothing, and nothing ever can. The supposedly ghetto politicians need more action and a lot less talking or inciting riots.

My Jimi Hendrix inspiration came from his *Cry of Love* album, which the song "Straight Ahead" is in. The album was released in 1971, soon after his death the previous September. The words to the song "Straight Ahead" are listed on the back cover of that album. Those words to me were written as though he is telling them from his grave. He writes and sings about being alone and needing help to make it or he may die. How spooky is that? The words to this song were very inspirational to me in 1971, the year I graduated from high school, and they always will be. I believe many of the verses to the song were about issues that he was trying to deal with before his death. Those issues were important to him before he died, and the same issues are just as important today for us. Many of these issues are incorporated in this book. He says a whole lot of people are coming down from drug highs. His own drug abuse problem eventually killed him. He says it is time to face reality about drugs and discrimination. He said we must all organize for the benefit of all, *which I am a proponent for*. He says to forget about the past issues (as in slavery) because things have changed. Today, we are so ingrained—with the many years of busing, most of our children in integrated schools, and multicultural everyday ethics—we *do not* need to be constantly reminded about slavery and oppression. He says we have to work together and *get over the past and work on issues,* not build separate, divisive groups. He also says our children need to be told the truth and not be told lies.

# 9.

# Religion

If you get anything out of reading this book, please understand that I am trying to present a simple case for good versus evil, rights and the right things to do. In Led Zeppelin's song "Stairway to Heaven" they allude to the fact that people have two paths they can take; however, there is plenty of time to switch from the path you are on. That is the way it is! If you are looking for some gray areas to choose as an easy way out of doing evil deeds, you are wasting your time. I usually do not wish anything bad for people, but in this case, if you mistreat your fellow brothers and sisters and are performing evil acts, there is a place for you.

For years there has been an easy explanation for how the game of football is played. It breaks down into two simple things: blocking and tackling. Many complex problems can be or solved in this simplified way. Start with the basic elements. Religion is no exception. Most of our religions are simply based on good versus evil.

In chapter 2, we discussed the differences between rights and the right things to do. I used the Bible's ten commandments as good practices for the right things and gave examples of their reciprocals—doing the wrong things. When using the reciprocal analogy, you may want to add this word to your personal vocabulary. The word is *pro-Semitic*. Yes, it is the opposite of that exceedingly popular word since 1932: *anti-Semitic*. I am a Christian and very pro-Semitic. I am especially now more than ever. The biggest reason will be discussed in more detail in our chapter on family. Please do not mind if I associate the use of *Semitic* with *Jewish*. I know there are differences. My point here is that practicing Jews typically have strong family ties. I would hope and pray that all the world's religions stress building strong, loving families. These are great starting points for teaching respect and discipline. Ancient and many present Eastern cultures still practice centering their cultures and values around strong family ties and respect for the elderly.

To mock or replace strong family upbringings with friends (to start with), then move it to social importance, or the media, then tie that into a government's role as more important than family, is laughable. If it were not for family most of us would not be here. Weakening families is a goal of some people today and the reciprocal of God's initial plans for Adam and Eve and the *garden made for them to play in*. For example, my definition for WOKE is War On Kindred Entities. Practicing it is at the center of the socialist trap to kill our family and cultural values and to start everyone's jail term to their government's absolute control of them. This is where government *is the end all be all!* This is their new world order.

One of my all-time favorite movies about good versus evil is *Cabin in the Sky*. This 1943 black-and-white film was recreated from the 1940 Broadway musical of the same name. It featured Ethel Waters, Eddie "Rochester" Anderson, Lena Horne, and Rex Ingram. Many of the scenes have Lucifer Jr. (the son of Satan himself) and the Lord's Angel doing a tug-of-war over a gambler that is trying to change his ways before death. In a similar take, when I was a child, I loved to read comic books. One of my favorites was Harvey Comics' *Hot Stuff the Little Devil*. The main character is Hot Stuff. He is an infant red devil that wears a diaper. Hot stuff tries to do bad deeds due to his lineage. Unfortunately for him, his own conscience often causes him to do good deeds instead.

This tug of war between good and evil is the same theme as the *Star Wars* movies. You know the story, going over to the dark side (evil) versus the force (good). I love all the *Star Wars* movies. It is unfortunate though that Holly-woke has to cast different groups of people, or different genders of people, as good or evil. Relative to Hollywood, I always want good to win over evil; it is the casting of the groups that have some political purpose in themselves that is a hateful, evil act. It is insensitive, divisive, and specifically targeting groups of people. I really believe they are initiating acts to specifically create a group of "scapegoats" to ostracize. They are using condition response. As mentioned in chapter 5 on the various media, they all seem to be doing this, being offensive to people and targeting them. *The point here is that media can and does move your feelings about good or evil, hate or color, and also affects your feelings about family and religion.*

In a National Geographic made-for-TV program on religion, the narrator, Morgan Freeman, showcased many of the world's religions. One of the religions was Zoroastrianism. He visited with groups of believers from California and Iran. Iran is where that religion was founded when the country was called Persia. The underlying theme of that religion is that people have good and evil within themselves, and that the evil within us *must be suppressed every day.* In the Christian faith, in the Lord's Prayer, or the Our Father, we say the words, "lead us not into temptation but deliver us *from evil.*" I suppose we could jokingly say that is an example of a hope and a prayer. However, seriously, doing the *praying* is the point, and not just a saying. We must lead ourselves to be delivered from evil.

The media for many years, through TV and movies, has portrayed evil in a way that makes it an abstract thing. In a sense, it is what some people do about their own inner evil, trying to mask it and dismiss it by using some left-handed attempt. Over the last two hundred years people have always tried to portray evil as an abstract thing. An example is Mary Shelley's *Frankenstein.* You may as well include Dracula and the Wolfman in one's abstract thinking about them being evil. When those evil creatures became less scary, we turned to Godzilla, and now the craze is zombies, vampires and dragons. Truth be told, it is *the people that do evil deeds* who are the most hazardous to humanity, like Hitler and Stalin. Well, I believe we are practicing our own internal evil because *we are dismissing it*. Speaking snarky or curt or being disrespectful to your parents is an evil act. Explain how being snarky, curt, and disrespectful has any good in it.

Previously we talked about doing the right things and the wrong things. We need to discipline ourselves into doing the right things. Again, rights versus the right thing to do. Even in our great push for rights there can be an underlying evil, selfish craving. As an example of this, we had slavery in this country because the southern plantation owners had rights and power. In this opioid epidemic we had doctors prescribing addicting drugs because they had rights and position. I should not have to explain the evils of Genghis Khan, Hitler, and the rest of those vile people. Remember that little antidote from the philosopher George Santayana. He said what our history teachers taught or should have taught. That is, "Those who cannot remember the past are condemned to repeat it." Unfortunately, we do it now more than ever. Rodney King on a television appearance discussed this issue. He pretty much said, "Can't we all get along?" Can we stop making it horrible for the older people and the kids too? Truer words were never spoken!

Recently a visitor to our country killed Americans because he said that we were *evil*. No, this is not a joke about the pot calling the kettle black. He murdered people, which is against most civilized nations' laws. How did he think his actions were good and not evil? We as nations must begin to lay the groundwork for decisions of what is good and what is evil. There should be no "get out of jail cards" for the freedom to *murder civilians*. Any group that does not embrace the whole breath of life and humanity should not be considered a religious organization. To go against life (taking the abortion rights issue out of the equation just for now) is a crime against humanity. We often have talked about the shortcomings of the United Nations and the World Health Organization today. These groups should have some kind of *legal definition* in their charters as to what is termed a "religion" (for humanity), and what is a "cult," and those who practice high crimes against humanity (human life) need to be swiftly held accountable. In another chapter I discuss governments; however, this is about religion and humanity.

I am a faithful believer in the visions that appeared at Our Lady of Lourdes (France) and Our Lady of Fatima (Portugal). The movies made for those events are some of my favorites. *Divine intervention is real.* I have a personal example of divine intervention. In the morning of November 2, in 2019, my mothers' nursing home called my brother and sister and I to come and visit my mother. Her attendants felt her time was at an end. She had been in terrible pain her previous two days and nights and had bouts of screaming with that pain. We all stayed with her that morning and most of the afternoon. I had to work later that afternoon, so I kissed my mother and told her that "she never looked lovelier." My job that afternoon was to drive a group of elderly residents to their 4:30 Saturday mass at their church. At 5:15 p.m., while waiting for them, I prayed at a fifteen-foot-high crucifix in the church's parking lot. I prayed for my mother's pain to stop and for God to comfort her. At 5:30, mass ended, and I drove everyone home. At about 6:00 p.m. my sister called my cell phone. She said my mother's nursing home called her and said our mom passed away at 5:15. That was precisely when I prayed to God to comfort her.

In the movie *Our Lady of the Fatima*, Lucia dos Santos is told in a vision by the Blessed Lady in Fatima that evil will come out of Russia and they should refuse to convert to Socialism. That was the time during the evil Stalin's regime. The evil did come out of Russia. It spread to Eastern Europe, China, Cuba, and then Venezuela, and now Brazil. The Soviet Socialist (leftist) regime was so evil, its military tried to kidnap Mikhail Gorbachev, their own premier (like our president) because he was allowing more freedoms (called *glasnost* in Russian). In America, we have a separation of church and state. That is the point here. Communist Socialism *does not* allow for religious freedoms. That is because their Socialist state, *one party,* is their one absolute religion, which is reliance on government for everything for everyone. Our churches and most religious organizations, which represent good by their deeds, know the *reciprocal* of good is evil. There is no wiggle room here folks. If evil people, for *their* own selfish reasons, run *your* country, that is what you get. An evil, selfish state.

You must remember that we are being monitored and recorded in every move we make today by the little pocket-sized LCD screens we have been "pushed into using." With these devices, our data could be monitored by Big Tech, the manufacturers of laptops, cell phones, TVs, and their programs. However, we easily dismiss that we are watched by God. People should not like it when Big Brother is watching, because it takes our freedoms and privacy away. Maybe that's why people also shy away from religion today? God is watching. Your record is clean when you are born. When you start doing bad things, evil things, they are recorded on YOUR record, whether at school, on the internet, or in public by somebody's camera. You need to have good pictures taken of all the good deeds you do. You need a snapshot of a clean bedroom, clean teeth, clean clothes and good manners. If your parents did not or would not encourage those simple practices, give yourself a good dose of self-discipline. You can keep those snapshots or images of your good behavior and live happily with them forever. *They help form your character* and that is what much of what this book is about.

For this chapter, my inspiration came from the songs "My God" and "I Saw God Today." "My God" was performed by Jethro Tull and sung and written by Ian Anderson. When I listen to that song it reminds me of what I learned in a saying as a youngster: "God helps those that help themselves." Of course the meaning was not for people to help themselves in life's pleasures or opportunities that may present themselves, but rather to identify one's own problems or issues in life and to take those all-important first steps for self-improvement. That part is where we are made in God's image.

"I Saw God Today" was sung by George Strait and written by Rodney Clawson, Monty Criswell, and Wade Kirby. In the song, George Straight sings about witnessing the birth of his brand-new baby daughter. Without mincing any words, he says that life itself is God's miracle. The song more or less mimics Jimi Hendrix's song "Straight Ahead" when he sang that the best love to have is "the love of life."

# 10.

# Men

In 2020 BC (before COVID), it was a lot easier to talk about how American men are behaving more selfishly than ever. However, as of this writing on May 11, 2020, I can see that many men have changed from that trend. I believe the COVID-19 pandemic has brought men closer together with their families (well, at least for now). I saw it happen this past Mother's Day weekend in 2020. The growing selfishness in men has begun to flatten the curve, as they say. Meeting your parents, or just talking with them on the phone for many of us, has a way of bringing us back to "the good ol' days." I know it did for my family. I could see it on my family's faces, especially on their mother's (my wife's) face. I could see how happy my wife was, and my children saw it too. They saw what it meant for our family to be together, especially through this lab-created nightmare of a pandemic. For me, this was the first year without my mother. As mentioned, she died in November 2019. I previously mentioned how unselfish she was, and I miss her, especially on this first Mother's Day without her.

You would think that being a man at the age of seventy-one, I would not have any trouble with writing about my observations of men. Well, it is not easy. I think a good start would be for me to talk a little bit about myself. I have tried to be a good father to my two daughters and two sons, and a good husband. You know the old adage, "happy wife, happy life." Believe me, all husbands should adhere to this practice. I believe I know when to stay firm with my opinions during domestic disagreements, when to leave them for another day, and when to just admit to being wrong.

I do have my circle of friends that I associate with. I see my friends or call them every now and then, but mostly my best friend is my wife. She cares for me, and I care for her. My other best friends are my children, whom we have shared so many great adventures with through our forty-five years of marriage together. The next old adage is the one about how you can only get out of something what you put into it. Believe me, that is the most important one when it comes to raising children. You can never give them enough attention because they are family, they are the future, and most of them, thank God, share your name.

I like an occasional glass of wine and prefer green tea to coffee, but I drink way too much coffee, and my wife often reminds me of it. Coffee keeps me awake, but it also brings out the Mr. Hyde in this Dr. Jekyll. I do not do drugs, but I take acetaminophen for my occasional headaches and ibuprofen for my sore body, especially after doing too much yard work. I am a retired public servant, but I have also worked part-time in the public sector. I still need that interaction with people, and my part-time job was perfect for that. My wife and I try to attend church weekly. Even though our children are married and out on their own, we still enjoy sitting with them at church when the occasions arise. I do not do Facebook or Twitter and try to avoid being on a computer or my smartphone more than I have to. I believe there is too much of life to observe in the real world, and men today are increasingly tied too tightly to their high-tech gadgets. Personally, I do not need to constantly crawl through an LCD screen like Alice peered through her looking glass (mirror) in the book *Alice's Adventures in Wonderland.* As we used to say in the '60s and '70s, "Get real, brother."

I believe many people today, not just men, do not want to accept the fact that life in America is tough. I believe it could be that they do not have perfect control of their lives. The appearance of being completely in control seems to be so important today. Man up. Life is tough, and you must do your part every day to smooth out those rough spots. So do not dismiss the hard facts of life. This country has the most freedom and is the greatest country in world, but understand, a lot of *good* people worked extremely hard, through some damn tough times, to get it there. Read an American history book. They have facts about our country and the heroes who helped build it. Work hard, guys. It is good for our country and proves we are winners and not a bunch of crybabies. You can have your fun, but after your work is done.

We talked about vices and distractions in chapter 6. For many men today, there are far too many. Consider the video games or pro sports on TV, or going to the sporting events. Why is there so much gambling today? Heaven only knows there is plenty of alcohol at these attractions, and that *is the distraction.* It seems men need to drink to be cool. If someone gets hungover, the homegrown recipe is to take an energy drink. That chemical combo will make you wacko. Incidentally, where are your children while you are occupying yourself with all these distractions that we just write off as entertainment? They are with your wife, naturally, and she is on the phone with her (divorce) lawyer.

My biggest problem with writing about men is that I feel I am ratting out my gender. For this chapter, I am going to rely on my unbiased scientific self. There is plenty of information about men everywhere—their life expectancy, drug abuse, erectile dysfunction (you hear the commercials), the divorce rate, and the amount that are contracting COVID, but that really is not what this is about. It is about my observations through my years in public service. I spent a good deal of my time in the scientific area of quality improvement, and that is how I am approaching this chapter.

I have had the pleasure in my career of working with many men from all kinds of backgrounds. Sometimes we would work and talk, but mostly we were able to talk at lunch. *It is very difficult today to assemble like that if you are working from home* (Viva la freedom of speech). We talked and enjoyed discussing the many issues of the day. My coworkers discussed their approach to work, marriage, families, education, finances, religion, and so on. Mostly though, they were happy because they were working and earning a livelihood. The most productive men in their workplaces were the ones who really enjoyed their work. They were lucky enough to have supervisors who were grateful that they were there and contributed to the organization in a positive manner. They were part of the team, no different than the team of players we watch in sports. As they say, the whole team of horses were all headed in the same direction. When you work with people like that, it makes you feel good. You feel good because you are visibly in reality, actively participating with work teams, and together usually headed in the same direction, the right direction, that you see as being successful. A good management team sees the successes of their employees in both their performance and employee attitudes. It is the essence of having a good personable relationship between an engaged management and their workforce.

I have met a few men, however, who did not want to work in a positive, productive manner. They were counterproductive, and that is like sabotaging the organization, or even a country. Those guys were plain miserable, and it made me miserable to hear them or be around them. I always explained to my four children to leave any job that you do not like. I told them that it is not fair to every other person in that organization to see you miserable at your job. Now, all four of them have careers they enjoy. You get out of life what you put into it. One should think that the organization *is paying its employees to do a full days' worth of work.* Some men would rather spite or even bite the hand that is feeding them. It is not just cheating on their commitment to do work, it is cheating our nation of its very important growth.

When a man gets out of high school, he is expected to "put his big boy pants on." He should become responsible for his well-being. He should, if he chooses marriage and family, be a willing party to help support them. He can expect some support from his parents per se, but now it is time to get focused on life and the big picture. Maybe teachers did not explain that most important point, probably because they had their own subjects they were responsible for, *but that is the point for education.* You and your teachers should have been planning for your own development. Men must face the facts that they are going to have to work to support themselves or their families and engage in our nation's needed growth. If they do not, everyone is going to feel the pain of not working one way or another. Everyone should understand that in our particular economic system, "we the people" expect you to do your fair share of working, paying taxes, and cutting our debts. If you can work but choose not to, you will be looked at as either disconnected or, at worst, lazy. I'm not trying to guilt you into working, but as my wife often says, "laziness trumps everything." Enjoy living in a free nation where you can choose your career or any job. In communist and socialist countries, they put you where *they* want to with *no regard* for your free thoughts about career choices.

People should choose careers they believe they will like and that have been shown to be somewhat *obtainable.* Enrolling in college and thinking anyone can achieve a six-figure computer programmer position may not be a good decision. The placement data says that is not likely to happen. There are only so many of those positions out there. Do not be fooled into thinking there is one for you. With that computer degree you will find yourself working at a cell phone store or as a computer repair tech in one of their lifelong apprenticeship programs. That will not remove that eighty grand or more of college financial aid debt that you will be carrying with you.

Men are so gullible today and lack basic, sound money-management skills. The data shows that they drink too much, *get impaired,* and put themselves in unhealthy and time-consuming habits. Conversely, many women have goals for brand-new homes, even right out of the gate after marriage. Perhaps both men and women should realize that a more practical approach is to purchase lower-priced homes that will create less debt. In the last century that was what most couples did, and it caused less financial stress in their marriages. Family finances is not some new fashionable trend. It is and always was a hardcore responsibility that lenders take very seriously no matter how much they smile at you when you sign up for those loans. There are many do-it-yourself home-improvement shows on TV today or other venues to teach about home remodeling. There is no better goal after high school than to focus on the American dream of owning your own home. It builds equity (sustainable value), is a large part of having financial security and safety, and historically takes people away from a continual life of renting, increased debt, and misery.

The music that inspired me to write this chapter came from the songs "Saturday Night's Alright (For Fighting)," sung by Elton John and written by Elton John and Bernard Taupin. I also received inspiration from the song "I'm A Man" performed by the Spenser Davis Group and written by Steve Winwood. In "Saturday Night's Alright" Elton John says he was undisciplined, only interested in getting drunk, looking for a date, and having a good time with his friends. Good luck with that headache tomorrow, Elton. However, with the doubling of alcohol consumption by people in my lifetime, I can only say I thought I had too many headaches back in my younger days. Spenser Davis pretty much mimics what Elton John sang. He adds, though, that he sees himself as rich and intellectual. The only thing that matters, though, is that he is addicted to loving women, but he is not going to commit to a long-term relationship (marriage).

These two songs tell a tale of how I observe American men today: too much entertainment, no discipline in their lives, and not committing to relationships and families—only to themselves. Those traits certainly do not help anybody but their selfish self. I can only hope that some men who read this chapter can turn the trend of increased alcohol and drug consumption and begin to "put their big boy pants on!"

# 11.

# Women

I often recall a nursery rhyme taught by my elementary school teachers many years ago. It is about what little boys and little girls are made of. However, for me the rhyme will always ring in my mind about what little girls are made of. It goes something like this:

What are little boys made of?
What are little boys made of?
Snips and snails
And puppy-dogs' tails,
That's what little boys are made of.

What are little girls made of?
What are little girls made of?
Sugar and spice
And everything nice,
That's what little girls are made of.

The one thing I did learn about little girls and women (after my wife and I nurtured our two girls and two boys) is that girls need their self-esteem raised more often than boys. I can relate to this from my experiences teaching children in a variety of programs. Psychologists have noted girls' self-esteem needs for years. Another observation is that girls and women "generally" tend to be more emotional regarding their decision making, and boys and men "generally" tend to be more rational (logical) in decision making. I'm okay with that, and I hope you are too! It is what it is. The truth does hurt some peoples' feelings sometimes, but when deciphering data, you need good factual data to formulate truthful conclusions, and those are the facts about men and women.

As a music fan, I also learned from James Brown's song "It's a Man's Man's Man's World." He sings that it is a man's world, but "it wouldn't be nothing, not one little thing, without a woman or a girl." Greater words were never spoken. Some women look at the history of our nation and see disparities in wages or other injustices in the workplaces. Some married couples see it in their marriages. Maybe that's why divorce is consistently on the rise (I discuss marriage in a later chapter). Partners should always add something positive to each other's life. The sacred bond of marriage is supposed to bring credence to the saying that two working together are better than one. The combined strength makes people better than if they tried to make it alone. The goal is to benefit both people while traveling through life together. Even if it is only to remove the feeling of loneliness. There can be nothing sadder than the hollowness of being lonely.

It is not too surprising that women have more self-esteem issues than men today. It is the added gender burden women face daily. Women also deal with the inherent notion that they are competing with other women. I think that is why women have the need to add to their arsenal of self-actualization tools (makeup, clothing, cars, homes, their jobs, social media, etc.). Buying things at times can be considered self-imposed perks for a person's accomplishments should they not be recognized by others. I do not see a problem with women's purchasing power to keep our economy growing, as long as they try to purchase *from local vendors and USA manufacturers*. It is a fact that women today make up about 75 percent of the purchasing power in America. I just hope and pray they are doing their homework before buying and reading the labels for where these items are made. Historically, Americans purchasing products made in the USA has led to higher wages for their employees. Let's keep our money in the family (our country) so to speak. Everyone should want to add higher paying jobs in their country. Since women make up 60 percent of all college graduates, that is of added importance.

Along with keeping up with the Joanies, women are continuously bombarded with an insurmountable amount of product advertising. Not just on over five hundred TV channels, but every time they pick up an electronic device or go into any store, specifically using their new best friend, the smart phone. When I see women today, I see that plastic leech attached to either their face or ear. I humorously call it "the face in the phone." That added anchor can be more of *a problem and not a solution*. The American Medical Association should identify these devices as not just fashionable, but rather as a social disease as habitual as smoking tobacco. The AMA should be lobbying for funding and developing treatment for all affected people.

I can remember watching some old classic movies from the 1940s and '50s and remembering the saying from those movies about door-to-door or traveling salesmen. The saying back then was to keep those salesmen from "getting their foot in the door." The salesmen's goal was to get housewives to buy vacuum cleaners, cleaning supplies, and healthcare products that even included snake oil. Hence the term "snake oil salesmen." Today what these sneaky salespeople do to get their foot into everyone's front door is to continually "knock" on all smartphone screens. This endless amount of advertising and messaging being thrown at women (and men too) inhibits their ability to take any time to focus on their objectives of the day. I had an occasion years ago to take a course in time management. With all these electronic messages thrown at people today, I believe that course should be a requirement taught in every high school in America. Consumer advocate Ralph Nader tried in the 1970s to make Americans more consumer conscious, but that message seems to have faded away. A person cannot continuously be on an electronic device with all that "chatter" and physically accomplish all of the necessities in their day's schedule. Incomplete tasks add up and can begin to add stress due to the disappointment of not completing them. With the important role that women have as product and merchandise buyers today, they without question are vulnerable consumers. The fact that women are such important consumers can add *additional stress* on them from advertisers. This is because women today are the *critical target market* for advertisers. This is a very broad subject and affects women in both professional and traditional roles. Women in the media should relish the importance that women have today. The limelight they are in should boost their self-esteem.

The dual role of working wives and mothers can lead to stress. With the elements of family, children, and work, and our media's constant intrusion on their cell phones, it must seem like they need another four hours in their day to get everything done. With all this going on, they have the added pressures of keeping up with their peers while watching their credit card debt go through the roof. Yes, women today are the target market with a *big bullseye* on their forehead.

For women working full time it is especially more difficult to plan and organize a household. Typically, including travel time, about nine hours out of their day is dedicated to a profession or a job. The few remaining hours of their day are used for meal planning and shopping. If they are blessed enough to have children, it must seem almost impossible to interact with them. Do not forget to add that schools expect parents to assist with homework. With electronic pad games children have today, this only *increases* the disconnect between young women and their mothers. Every time I hear the Beatles song "Got to Get You Into My Life" I think about parenting. After describing what women deal with every day I am glad I am a man.

The women with the most difficult challenges to overcome today are the minorities. When my editor asked me who *my target market is for this book,* I told him anybody that would listen. The truth is I do have a priority list of readers that I believe will find this book beneficial. It begins with the neediest. They are women of color living in poverty or never-ending debt. Other than our children, they are our society's most vulnerable for exploitation. What has disturbed me for many years is that our impoverished women in America have become the most ostracized on one hand, exploited on the other, and dis-R-E-S-P-E-C-T-ed...period. For example, one can hear this misogyny in some rap music. These women of color are usually single parents, many of them reduced to living in crime-riddled ghettos and feeling trapped in a lifestyle with no chance for change and no way out. Additionally, they feel that no one understands their plight. The worst part is because they are being classified as a minority. Adding insult to injury, due to the quality, or lack thereof, in our public school education in larger cities, they may have a misperception of the term *minority*. *Minority* is a term used by our government to mean the ratio or percentage of the whole population (like 10 percent Hispanic). It is not to be taken to be mean a lesser value of person or group of people. Everyone is intitled to the same rights as everyone else in the United States. The Equal Rights Amendment has been ratified in thirty-eight of our fifty states, and in most states with large, impoverished cities. I do not believe the inner-city schools are teaching those important principles. That is what it truly means to be a minority: every citizen's rights; historically, America's importance in the world as a beacon for democracy and personal liberties; and *their duty to maintain it!* Without knowing those basic principles, it is no wonder why today's inner-city women may harbor a distrust for some people in our government. Our country has thousands of stories of how minorities with lower economic means have succeeded and become famous. *All women need to know that the total of all American people support them and want them to succeed...period!* There is no need to exploit any woman in our country today. It is shameful.

Make no mistake, women are definitely different than men. Anyone, even without 20/20 vision, can see the physiological differences. Our body parts alone attest to that fact. We already know about women's issues with PMS, hormonal changes, birth defects, breast cancer, and the list goes on and on. Women have enough issues to deal with without constantly being reminded that it is a man's world. It is not a man's world, because it would be as James Brown sang: It wouldn't be nothing, not one little thing, without a woman or a girl.

The music that inspired me to write this chapter came from the songs "Stairway to Heaven," performed by Led Zeppelin and written by Jimmy Page and Robert Plant, and "The Girl from Ipanema," sung by Astrud Gilberto and written by Antonio Carlos Jobim and recorded by Stan Getz. "Stairway to Heaven" was a song I sang with the rock group I was in. So it has a special meaning for me. Now when I hear it, it reminds me that women have 75 percent of the purchasing power in America today. I think that is great for our economy to keep it going, but I wonder if they are paying attention to where the products they are purchasing are being manufactured. It is vitally important to keep as much of our money and resources as possible here in the United States so we can begin to produce higher-wage jobs and sustain a strong manufacturing base. *Those higher-wage jobs are for every woman's children to earn!*

Every time I hear the song "The Girl from Ipanema" it causes me to have a mental picture of a sunny beach with girls walking by with their newly purchased fashionable swimwear and the young men eyeing them up. I started this chapter with a nursery rhyme about how girls are sugar and spice and everything nice. So, ladies, do not ruin that great old nursery rhyme. We all want that vision and impression of you. I have two daughters, and my 20/20 vision tells me that you are hopeful that your daughters will fit into the theme from that nursery rhyme.

# 12.

# Dating, Relationships, and Premarital Activities

The term *dating* in this chapter refers to couples, historically or naturally, trying to develop romantic/intimate relationships. It is about couples going out to theatres, cinemas, or other entertainment venues and hopefully enjoying the pleasure of each other's company. I have watched this process happening through the years, and having four married children, I have seen a lot of it. Dating over the past one hundred years was never supposed to have any prerequisites. It was to go out and have some fun together and share some interests. Unfortunately, with the pressures our adolescents face regarding sex and how entertainment and media outlets portray it, it affects the intended spirit of how couples can just talk and laugh together. That should be the intention of the date. After the date, hopefully everyone will have good memories of it.

Dating has changed so much through the years. In the nineteenth century and earlier, it was customary for young couples to have chaperones. I can recall when my eldest daughter was a student at Kent State University and lived on and near the campus, she would tell me that she went out with friends on the weekend. This did not bother my wife and I too much, because we knew she was involved in religious ministries and other quality activities on campus. She never said she had a steady boyfriend. She had a group of young men and women friends that would go out and socialize together. I believe many of the students' parents wanted their children to develop a sense of independence. The TV series *Friends* may have created that culture. For my children, college was a way to view how people their age acted socially.

My wife and I talk about the subject of dating all the time. We both agree that we are glad we dated at a time when there was not as much pressure being placed on adolescents. I feel bad for adolescents because of the pressures society puts on them. How can you go to high school or college, where the priority is to hopefully crack open books and learn and still develop socially? All the movies made today seem to be made only for specific viewer ratings. Young adults look at the movie ratings before attending any movies. If it is not rated X, they usually will not view it. That is a sad situation, because there are so many movies and documentaries with invaluable social messages. Even the TV commercials create social pressures. There are too many male enhancement commercials. Even standing in the grocery store checkout lines can be another stressful adventure for some of us. If you have young children with you, the parents many times would like to turn the tabloid magazines around, or block them so their children do not see the "newsworthy" headlines and photos. *For my family*, TV channels or programs that offer no advertisements, or DVD movies, create less social stress.

When talking about sex and dating, how do families deal with it? With the ever-increasing rate of divorce today, how can parents give guidance to their children? I believe they cannot or will not, because parents may appear hypercritical when asked about sex or dating. Their children could respond to their parents by saying, "Who are you to tell me about the person I'm dating? Look at your failed marriage (marriages)." That is a tough pill to swallow. However, parents *must* deal with it.

Recently, I overheard some elderly female friends that were in their eighties discussing their grandchildren. One of them said that their married grandchildren were having some serious problems. One of them went on to say, "They are not children anyone. Who am I to give my opinion?" The other lady nodded her head as though in agreement. Since they were my friends as well, I interjected. I gave them a quote from the movie *There's No Business Like Show Business*. I told them what Ethel Merman said in the movie. Ethel played a Vaudeville show-business mother, and her son was played by Donald O'Connor. He left their family's show business for years after a disagreement and never left a trace of where he was. When he finally returned to his family, Ethel said, "You know, you worry about your kids from the time they are born until the day you die." I explained to my friends that they are their children's parents forever. As parents and grandparents, and having more knowledge and experience about such things as marriage and family, it is both their right and the right thing to do to give their children advice through the good times as well as the bad times. Whether their children accept their advice or not, that is their prerogative.

There is far too much emphasis on sex today, being "cool," and trying to establish a mainstream society to turn everyone into robotic Stepford wives. That is in reference to the 1970s TV series *The Stepford Wives*. The plot for the series was that the women in a small New England community were gynoids, or programmed female androids, created by the males of the community. Who wants to be a controlled robot anyway? What "they," the government and media, never mention to our adolescents is that God has placed some *dangerous equipment* in the hands of an *indifferent generation*. Reproductive organs were designed for couples to use after marriage, or at least at a point where couples are mature enough to *respect each other*.

I cannot tell you how much I appreciate the advertisements on TV about respecting women. We often read about the pressures that were placed on actresses by high profile movie producers for sexual favors. We also learned about high society people using escort services that cultivate minors for "entertainment" purposes. That disrespect is not about boys being boys, or girls being girls. It is about respecting one another's body and mind. It is about not using physical, mental, and sexual abuse. This chapter is about developing respectful relationships with friends that will last a lifetime. Be kind and considerate, and the USA and the world will have many more civilized people in it.

For this chapter, my inspiration came from the song "Que Sera Sera." *Que sera* is Spanish, and therefore, the song was meant to mean "whatever will be, will be." It was sung by Doris Day and written by Jay Livingston and Ray Evans. This song was often played on radio stations in the mid-1950s. It is considered the thirty-second best hit from that decade. It was a time when people learned to let go of the situations or things they could not control, because it leads to frustration. It is important for people to have faith. It is so positive to do so. Looking at events that seem to be a forever circumstance is shortsighted. Things change in our lives and in our world and always will. Our world has had the benefit of people throughout history working tirelessly to help make it a better place. I believe they were given a gift or the inspiration to do so.

However, the phrase "whatever will be, will be" has a whole new meaning when considering the way that artificial intelligence can and probably has affected "natural" occurrences. What I call natural occurrences are anything left alone to happen naturally without someone or something, like AI, analyzing the event's data. After the occurrence, interested parties can have meaningful cues introduced into the data. This ultimately modifies the occurrence's reporting for the benefit of that interested party. Do not misunderstand me, technology has helped predict many things, for example, when to take our automobiles in for predictable or preventable maintenance. Department stores and other company use AI to track sold items and predict automatic reorder points. However, AI can be a double-edged sword. The fact is that data can be manipulated, copied, then pasted and reentered and therefore can negate the accuracy of the data. An example would be if a computer were programmed to scan something, a word, a name, or even a vote, and be programmed to delete it, it would in essence negate the original intended purpose of computers (being a speedy electronic tabulation machine for numbers/data etc.). "The scarier part is when AI is used to program programs. AI could infer that human interjections, which are not infallible, can cause errors in programs and therefore (humans) may need to be eliminated."

The absence of laws or regulations preventing any manipulations *should be a major concern for everyone*. We depend on real data or information to make our *human* decisions. Using tampered data to "tip the scales" to benefit special interest groups does not help with searching for the truth. Modified information is contaminated information. "My acronym for that is MOF, manipulation of facts." Basically, the information can be lies. The interested groups receive their paid-for "self-fulfilling prophecy" and leave the rest of the populace dumbfounded. Therefore, the term "que sera, sera," or "whatever will be, will be," although true in the 1950s, is not factual in the twenty-first century.

When you meet an interesting person that you would like to date or just spend some time with, talk a lot about your interests and their interests at length. Try to "get to know" their character. Ask yourself, "Is this a person I want to spend a lot of time with and to know better?" Are they true to themselves, or just playacting through your time together? Have you caught them lying about anything? You should be able to spot a phony or fake person imitating perhaps some famous person. After you learn to trust each other more I believe you will find, if nothing else, you made the beginnings of some important memories together.

# 13.

# Marriage

I would hope that every American is as fortunate as my wife and I to be in a relationship as we have for over forty-seven years. We met in college between classes. We dated and had our little disagreements through dating, but we came out of those experiences with a better understanding of each other. When I asked my wife to marry me it was because I knew I had met a truly honest and transparent person. I realized I had met a person who was wise beyond her years. She was eighteen years old, and I was twenty-two. We really enjoyed each other's company, and we both knew that this was something that could last forever. We fell in love. I will never forget the expression on my father-in-law's face when I asked him if I could marry his daughter. He looked at me, taken totally by the surprise, and said, "We better go in and let Dorsay (my wife's mother) know about this." Well, the rest was history.

We had a marriage engagement lasting ten and a half months. The next thing we knew we were engrossed with wedding plans and all that pressure that goes along with it. We did not have a wedding planner. We did not have a textbook titled *Wedding Planning for Dummies*, nor a computerized project management program to track our progress. It was not so painstakingly hard on me. I was going to be the groom. My three biggest jobs were to get measured for my tuxedo, buy the liquor, and make sure I knew when to say "I do" at church. I also had to make the plans for us to meet with our pastor and go through all the pre-wedding training. The training, called Pre-Cana, was greatly beneficial for us, and I suggest that all couples attend similar pre-marriage counseling before their marriage. There really *is no substitute for experience* from people, including your parents, about marriage to keep newlyweds from pitfalls and eventual failure. Later in our marriage my wife and I worked along with about a half a dozen other married volunteers from our church who helped others in their Pre-Cana classes.

The wedding planning was a real double-edged sword for my wife. There were halls to rent, caterers to call, invitations to write, wedding dresses to pick out, and many phone calls to make. That was only part of the planning. Everyone says success is all about completing the details. Believe me, there were plenty for our wedding. My suggestion, due to the stress of the wedding planning itself, is that you make this a once-in-a-lifetime event. Yes, you can hire a wedding planner. However, I believe most newlyweds would prefer to have the money that is spent on a wedding planner and use it as the down payment on their first home.

From my observations about weddings and marriage, people, or should I say couples, put too much emphasis on the wedding event and not enough on their marriage. They learn that weddings are very expensive but fun. They look at all the photos from other people's weddings and see how friends got drunk and said and did some outrageously funny things. We did at ours! Weddings make you feel good…FOR A DAY! Or maybe you remember the hangover you had the day after.

Marriage should be looked at as a long voyage. It is intended for a lifetime. It is where you find couples understanding they are in a marriage *operation* and now have big responsibilities. Together they must put everything into it, and good planning for the marriage is a must. The rose-colored glasses many times have to be traded in for safety glasses, because it can be a rough ride.

Marriage is dynamic; there is no crystal ball showing the future. In chapter 3, "Your Character, Our Country, and Our Culture," I discussed a line from the movie the *Sound of Music*. It is "nothing can come from nothing." You learn marriage is a WORK IN PROGRESS every day. It is a serious commitment. That is the deal. There should be a printed section on the bottom of every marriage certificate that says it is a performance-based contract. Couples have entered into a legal partnership, much like any business partnership. Like a business it is intended for *growth*. The combined strengths of two people are stronger, or meant to be stronger, than one. There are no days off. If you do not fulfill your obligations to your marriage contract there are very expensive consequences.

When trying to find any "me" or selfish time, it can be very difficult. It is a 24/7 agreement (twenty-four hours a day, seven days a week) when considering the most important job *is to support your marriage*. Each partner should understand that there is a time for work and a time for play. Playtime is very important for each other though. Like any businesses, people become stressed out. However, those relaxation times may prove to be harmful should they become too expensive and selfish fetishes. Some activities, like the time spent on "MyFace" or the internet, or shopping or gaming, many times prove to be *counterproductive* to a marriage. The question is how much your playtime will affect your marriage. Those activities tend to waste valuable time and can blow the family's budget. Couples *need* a budget because of their mutual responsibilities; they need a vision or plan for financial security.

If you think weddings are expensive, the reverse weddings—the event where you go downtown to see the divorce lawyers—are even more expensive. You won't need to do much planning. Most states in our country have made the process of divorce prearranged, like a canned computer program, and you are escorted through that process by the lawyers. Believe me, having four children, all having been married, I know a few things about wedding expenses and divorce costs. A very good friend of mine and mentor that was contemplating a divorce humorously advised, "It is cheaper to keep her!"

When I think about marriage, three songs keep ringing in my ears. They are the inspiration for this chapter. They are "Waiting for a Girl Like

You," "Running Against the Wind," and "Me and Bobby McGee." Each of the three songs remind me of phases that marriages may go through. "Waiting for a Girl Like You" is sung by Lou Gramm of the rock group Foreigner and written by Lou Gramm (Grammatico) and Mick Jones. Lou Gramm sings about how he has been looking for and waiting to find the girl of his dreams. He eventually does. I really believe that patience is a virtue, and it pays off in the long run.

"Running Against the Wind" is a song written by Bob Seger and performed by Bob Seger and the Silver Bullet Band. It is a tale of love and promises. Unfortunately for the singer, it tells how his marriage ended with a separation. The singer tells how he wishes he could have been more prepared for the grind and hardship that can come with marriage. As he found himself more engrossed in his job and supposed friends, he fell further from his home and his real happiness. I believe that can be said by many former couples.

The song "Me and Bobby McGee" is sung by Janis Joplin and written by Fred L. Foster and Kris Kristofferson. Janis Joplin sings about her relationship with Bobby McGee. In that relationship she says that just feeling good was good enough for her and Bobby McGee. Unfortunately, because of their wandering around America, they lost hold of their love for each other; however, she does hope he will find the happiness in whatever he was looking for. Their relationship was another example of a couple not knowing each other's goals. However, they had some great times and fun together, and she remembers those moments and has no regrets, has good memories of Bobby McGee, but now is left alone.

# 14.

# Family and Parenting

Most people know that there is nothing more important that will affect our world's future than our children. Even before their K-12 education they *may* receive is the parenting they *must* receive. Must receive? Why is that? If the future of the world is at stake, a solid foundation for infants is a must. I made my point and will give positive advice on parenting and family building.

My wife and I had the pleasure and responsibility to raise four children from childbirth to adulthood. For us parenting began during our discussions about it during our dating and continued into our engagement, and we still discuss it as we care for our grandchildren. When we dated, we discussed how many children we should have. I came from a family with an older sister and brother. Along with my father and mother, I loved them all. My father and mother were born in Cleveland, Ohio, and both had large families. I was blessed to have all my uncles and aunts living in our neighborhood. My wife was the oldest of six children. Her father and mother were dedicated to their family. Her father was from Patton, Pennsylvania. He had four sisters, and I had the pleasure of meeting his mother and father. Her grandfather was a retired coal miner, and that career had him affected by what is called black lung disease. My wife's mother came from a family of fourteen children. Her mother was raised in Gallitzin, Pennsylvania. That is where my wife's father and mother met. It was at a local roller-skating rink.

My wife and I love children. While a teenager, my wife had the dubious honor of being the neighborhood babysitter. She always enjoyed watching children and took that responsibility seriously. She still takes childcare seriously as she and I watch our grandchildren, which is almost daily. My role in parenting was to be the supporting husband, and I tried to be the all-important breadwinner. Our jobs were to keep the wheels from failing off our family's adventure. I learned many things from her about parenting. She knew how demanding it was for a family to function effectively. Two parents are needed. God help those people, and most importantly the children, who are denied that necessity. Incidentally, my wife worked as a childcare professional. In 2010 she received a national award for her teaching efforts and abilities.

## BE A GOOD LISTENER

There is an unbelievable responsibility that goes with parenting. Most important is the direct personal engagement with your children and discussions about their activities. This means *you* need to be a good listener. Every time I hear the Beatles song "Got to Get You Into My Life," it reminds me how much children want YOU and *need* YOU in their lives. My wife often says, "No one wants to be ignored." That is especially true for children. To some extent, children are like computer systems that have practically unlimited operating system storage. Like a sponge to water, they actively soak up information and view all activities in their surroundings. That includes what you do or don't do! If you, the parents, are not the ones providing for their surroundings and well-being, they will be "programmed" by others. In chapter 2 we discussed your character and that nothing comes from nothing and never can. With parenting comes your chance to contribute to your child's future, which in turn enhances your future, our country's future, and reshapes our world's future.

## EMBRACING THE ROLE AS A PARENT

In chapter 12 on dating and relationships I mentioned the conversation I heard between two elderly women who were grandparents. They were discussing their married children's marital problems. I overheard them saying, "They are not children anymore. Who am I to give my opinion?" I explained to my friends that they are their children's parents *forever*. As parents and grandparents, having more knowledge about such things as marriage and family, it is both your right and the right thing to do to give your children advice through the good times and the bad times. I gave those *grandparents* advice, and now I am advising all parents to do the same thing. You are your children's parents *forever*. Take up the responsibility that inherently has been bestowed upon you as a parent. You must nurture, teach, and lead as a role model and advise them on important things like morality and ethics. As a parent there is no time to be "the cool" parent and be their friend as well. Too much is at stake. Do not be steered into believing the latest buzz words by lazy parents that use trite sayings like *helicopter* (hovering) or *lawn mower* (clearing obstacles) *parents*.

A child's behavioral development many times mimics other children's behavior. Your children see both the good behavior and bad behavior in their play groups as youngsters and in their peer groups later in life. Help children understand that what they do affects them *and* others and how others perceive them. They need examples of how good deeds help to comfort people or make them feel good when needed. They need to know these are good, positive acts of kindness, and conversely need to know what are evil acts that have a negative effect on people and emotionally hurt them. You are the influencing factor in their character building. My mother once said that "No matter what, children will turn out okay." My mother was a modest woman. She never gave herself enough credit for being a working mother who tried to make all kinds of ends meet during some hard times. My mother may have sung along with Doris Day's "Que

Sera Sera" (whatever will be, will be); however, she practiced the belief that you only get out of life what you put into it.

## PARENTAL GROWTH

In 1946, Dr. Benjamin Spock, a very popular pediatrician, wrote a book titled *Baby and Child Care*. It sold over 500,000 copies and was a bestselling book in the twentieth century. His methods were liberal if not radical for that time. [1]He said, "Love and enjoy your children for what they are, for what they look like, for what they do, and forget about the qualities that they don't have. // The children who are appreciated for what they are grow up with confidence in themselves and happy. They will have a spirit that will make the best of all the capacities that they do have, and all of the opportunities that come their way". From that statement, I believe he was emphasizing the simplicity of continual love for them, as themselves, because it will make parenting easier and less stressful for the parent and child. Love has a way of doing that. In essence, take a deep breath and relax, because everything will be okay. Somewhat a "que sera sera" attitude. Receiving childcare experience from mothers or others is important. However, equally important is to be a student in new methods that have been shown to be effective with children. This is a different time and environment from when Dr. Spock was writing. For example, young girls do not play with dolls as often as they once did. Therefore, continue to learn from your trusted mentors (family), but do not stop there. There are books and magazines that have many good articles by knowledgeable professionals.

It may not be scientifically accepted, but I believe there are inborn *motherly feelings* that occur between a mother and her children. We see that bond between almost every animal on earth. There are shared tears when children are in pain. *Mothers do not dismiss those inner feelings.* Your children may need that natural behavior of yours in dealing with some matters.

For older children, Boy Scouts and Girl Scouts have proven to have positive effects on children's social skills. The scouting programs have crafts and group activities that give children the needed tactile skills that electronic tablets can never deliver.

Children should be in *at least one* school or organized sports activity. It helps to keep them physically active (especially *during pandemics* when schools have mandated virtual classroom sessions). Sports can also prevent the potential for obesity. Organized sports isn't just about exercise and socializing with friends. It teaches children the importance of interdependence while working toward successful results.

There can be nothing more stabilizing in a child's life than having them accompany you when attending places of worship (churches or temples, etc.) and the routine of religious practices. Religious freedoms are protected by our constitution. The freedom to assemble (hopefully peacefully) is also on that list. Our constitution's framers may not have known what the future would hold for our nation, but they knew how important religious beliefs were and witnessed how powerful nations and groups have tried to eliminate them. I've watched children from a variety of religions unbiasedly play and work together. They are children and do not have any predisposed prejudices. Most religions understand human frailty. Many teach that the love of God (or gods) and fellow man is the foundation to their religion. Those differences between people can never shake their foundations. Most religions also have the fundamental belief in helping the less fortunate. Acts of kindness toward others by parents cement the importance of serving the less fortunate over selfish behaviors. I do not mean placing cans of food in boxes, but physically helping others, such as volunteering to work at hunger centers. Those acts are the real ones, *not the virtual ones*. Those interactions plant the seeds of love and kindness that most religions support. Important acts of providing nourishment or unused clothing to improve health and safety needs demonstrate kindness. People helping people puts joy on impoverished faces, and those pictures last a lifetime. There is enough bad news today, and your children will see positive acts that help others, not harm them. Our ancestors believed in and worshiped a higher being than ourselves. One of my favorite rock groups, Spirit, released an album titled *The Family That Plays Together Stays Together*. That title was actually taken from a trite saying, "The family that prays together stays together." I believe that playing music together and praying together are both acts that elevate family life.

## THE FAMILY PLAN

What are your parenting and family plans now? How are you going to be actively involved in your children's lives? How are you going to manage your time for that? After forty-seven years of marriage and over forty years of parenting, I learned something. Know that *your* family is *your business* with *your name* on it. To be an effective and not a dysfunctional family, it needs to be managed and be *business-like*. The five basic principles for effective management are: planning, organizing, staffing, leading, and controlling.

Businesses and effective families use management principles. The first thing a business knows is that growth is essential, and it cannot grow without an understanding of its income, expenses, and operational needs. A business will go bankrupt if their expenses exceed their income. Loans and borrowing with interest rates only add to debt, which kills growth. It is the same for families. Couples have to look at their combined income and their expenses. Those expenses are apartment rent or home loan payments, car, utilities, food, clothing, and healthcare expenses. Running a household by the seat of your pants only works for the rich and famous. I am going to tell you this fact and take it as the gospel truth. A bank or financial institution does not care if your home loan with them falters. If you go into default on your home loan and cannot make the payments, you will be evicted. The lending institutions will financially break even when your former home is liquidated. They did, however, benefit, as most leaders do, by the loan interest payments you made to them. It is up to you to get a sustainable home loan that benefits you. Saving for a large down payment for a home makes good economic sense. Understand that investing in homes and property is like a savings account and money in the bank. The equity usually grows, and your investment is *not a wasted expense*. Homes become a psychological "safe house" for families, a fortress of solitude, so to speak.

A home in a safe neighborhood does offer a sense of security for a family. Your neighbors are in the same boat as you are. They pay taxes for services to upkeep the area like school systems, road repairs, garbage collection, and police protection. It's a wonderful feeling to know your neighbors are mostly like you, trying to make ends meet and trying to provide a good home and life for their children. In our neighborhood, most neighbors help each other when they can.

Home and property expenses inherently occur. However, most families get into economic trouble when unnecessary expenses—the *wants*, not the *needs*—occur. When you let pushy advertisers run up your debt, your family's stability starts to run on shaky ground. Homeowners trying to maintain a family must establish a family budget and stick to it. Salespeople today know how to have you spend your income. It is worse when you spend money that you have not even earned yet (credit cards).

Parents make up the initial family planning. They also are the leadership, organizing, and controlling factors. A major controlling factor is the leadership needed regarding time management. Not managing your time effectively will affect everyone in your family, especially the family's budget. As the saying goes, "time is money." A family's expenses require incomes to *overcome* those expenses. Decisions about those incomes many times are made on the fly (a sudden loss of a job, etc.). I know this is a hard pill to swallow; however, working and having a job is essential to acquire income to pay for the family's needs. Career changes that are wants and not needs, if not planned on before having children, can become costly expenses. For example, the expense for childcare if required for a career change can be as expensive as the income from that career. You also have to consider the educational or training costs for that career. Additionally, there may be intangible costs from the time away from the family to consider. Many families have been broken up by those advertisements about going back to college and getting degrees. If the job market is not conducive to hiring your degree program, you lost out on the college expense and the time away from your family. With the job market situation as it is, and the investment being three times the minimum wage rate, it will not pay for itself. Again, career paths should have been planned and long established before building a family, or at least after most of the children have carved out their own careers and your home mortgage loan has been paid off.

The family's staffing grows as the children grow. Delegating tasks and duties are a necessity. They are necessary *so parents can lessen their load.* Children must learn the responsibilities of a family and the interaction involved. Learning by doing is the best tool for kids to learn from. Children should be watching *you* do the task first, and not sitting down glued to their electronic gadgets as you do the work. Have them work with you as you teach them to do it. Each task delegated gives you more time to control your schedule (time). Crosby, Stills, Nash, and Young had a song, "Teach Your Children." Sounds like great advice.

We mentioned about your children being on their electronic devices. Our electronic age was supposed to make our society more productive. If playing games on them makes us more productive, *I haven't seen it.* You must not only monitor the amount of time your children are on their electronic devices and television, but more importantly the programs they are on and watching. My grandchildren bring their tablets over to our home when we are watching them for their parents. The first thing they ask me is to connect them to the internet. My response is, "The internet?"

The internet is the most crooked road to ride on since stagecoaches tried to run though the badlands. Our internet is not *clinical* or problem free! If there are not pre-approved games on their devices by the parents, learn to say no to any internet connection. For television programming, please watch those programs with them. If they are inappropriate, you are the adult with the remote control in your hand. Most of these programs are all about *cool* over *family*. The National Geographic programs probably never looked so good to you after seeing some of the children's network TV programming.

## CONCLUSION

The coaches with successful winning teams in sports and businesses instill an unselfish, relentless attitude. Those successful teams set goals and benchmarks. They gather the resources and tools necessary to achieve those goals. They continuously measure their team's achievements and recognize and discuss their successes with them (as praise). Regressions are openly discussed, and corrective actions are made from brainstorming. Successful families must do these same things. Successful teams many times emulate other successful teams. Why reinvent the wheel? When you build your family, you are building a part of your country. You are designing it in your image, your family's image. Just as cultured pearls are made to be flawless, so can our families be polished and refined. While building your family, you may also want to look at the broken ones. What are they doing wrong? The data suggests that the problems of rising debt, alcohol, and drug abuse are the culprits. Also wasting too much time buying too many wants instead of needs. The most important thing to recognize is the importance of interdependence among family members and the love you share by getting into each other's lives because you care for each other. Families understand about walking a mile in each other's shoes. Basically, share stories of the day and take an interest in what each other's plans are.

For this chapter, my inspiration came from the songs "Having My Baby" and "Mother's Little Helper." "Having My Baby" was written by Paul Anka and sung by Paul Anka and Odia Coates. "Mother's Little Helper" was written by Keith Richards and Mick Jagger and performed by the Rolling Stones.

In the song "Having My Baby," Paul Anka praises his partner for the sacrifice that she makes in giving nine months of her "normal" life to carry a baby in the hopes of them having a child. Paul Anka sings that there is no better way to show how much she must love him.

In "Mother's Little Helper" it is almost the reversal of the song "Having My Baby." The mother in the song only complains about her children and how they are wearing her down. For her relief she takes drugs to calm herself down. This is absolutely not the right thing to do. The old saying goes that an ounce of prevention is worth a pound of cure. The mother described in this song probably should not have had children if she was going to end up being a drug addict. There are preventative measures for couples to not have children. Medically, hysterectomies for women and vasectomies for men. These procedures prevent pregnancies that *make the whole* Roe v. Wade *discussion needless for some.* For women, the medical procedure eliminates the potential dangers of having children, because *not all pregnancies go smoothly.* About between 70 to 75 percent of human conceptions fail and do not lead to childbirth. *Make no mistake, there are dangers for women during pregnancy.* I will not discuss birth defects associated with pregnancies. That topic is too emotional for discussion. The costs for hysterectomies for women and vasectomies for men *should be covered under certain healthcare plans.* To date most vasectomies for men are reversible. However, hysterectomies for women are not. For adults that cannot have children on their own, they should consider adopting or becoming a foster parent. In the USA there are around 120,000 children each year available for adoption. *There is no more noble act than adopting a child.*

# 15.

# Love, Hate, and Divorce

**LOVE**

In the chapter on dating and relationships I discussed the feelings when couples are in love. Believe me, love can hit you like a brick. However, is the partner you are choosing ready for a long-term relationship? Are you ready to love each other *forever*? Maybe you are just going to plan a quick trip to Las Vegas, get married, and tell all your friends on "MyFace," "Hey look, see, we are adults now." Maybe you are married, knowing marriage is only a legal thing. It could be like getting a fishing license, not knowing how to fish. In that case getting married would be a childish thing, not an adult thing. If either of you are not certain that this is a forever thing, my advice is, do *not* get married. You can stay friends, and I hope you do. In time you both may see how you miss each other's company and really feel the *loss of love* for each other. You may understand that you are now ready to measure up to marriage. Remember that there is a difference between rights and the right thing to do.

Being in love and wanting to keep that "fire" burning is a process. It is an adult process in your journey together. If you really love each other you should instinctively want to safeguard each other from harm. You should always talk about your love for each other *to each other*. It's nice to hear it, right? Discuss how you first met and why you met. Talk about all the good times you had. However, as the saying goes, words of love may not win a person's heart. Many famous people have similarly spoken that statement. It goes like this: "Deeds, not words." Couples should take vacations or time off together because it keeps the "fire" burning. That is how to re-kindle your love. Those special times together will tell you both that the little monetary sacrifice for this event is the proof that your love is cemented in deeds and not just words. Therefore, clear your calendars and get ready to focus on this time together. It is a time for no distractions and dedicated to each other. Believe me, if you do this, the memories will last a lifetime for you.

If there are obstacles in your way that may jeopardize your love, discuss them. We know there are mean, envious people out in our world who hate to see people happy and will interfere with your relationship. Usually these people are just miserable and want to pass that feeling on. As they say, "misery loves company."

The most important thing that couples in love should always have is respect for each other. Take the time to observe each other's behavior. How can you have respect for anyone you if you do not know them? Is this a *real* person? In the 1960s and '70s we would call phony people "plastic." If you were deceitful or dishonest and "plastic" at some time in your life it may be time to modify your behavior. You may have to give this advice to your partner, hopefully early on in your relationship. If you want your love to be true, you need to understand that *you* need to be true. Your love will never work out if you are not true to each other. That behavior is the foundation for respecting each other. Being true to each other *leads to respecting each other*.

You may not have noticed but God has placed dangerous equipment in and on the bodies of women and men. You need to be aware of those dangers and think about the consequences when they are misused. People that practice being true do not change their partners like people change their socks. The amount of time and emotion that couples share with each other tells you that you don't have to go looking for love. You are in a continuous construction stage with it. Should you have children I do not think you would want them to remember you as "the unfaithful rambler." Your character is your reputation; do not take any steps backward in your character. The forward steps become much harder to take, if not impossible. Your actions show your character and your reputation. Even your clothing can send signals about the commitment to your marriage. Are there lots of clothes in your closet? Fashionable clothing is popular but should not be too revealing. God is watching and recording your acts. Even worse, Big Tech and everyone else is snapshotting a record of you.

## HATE

My wife and I always told our children never to use the word *hate*. As in, "I hate that person." There are people that do some terrible, evil things to other people. If they have affected you in some manner you must be stronger than they are. Please try and understand that they are weak or sick and have pity on them. Two wrongs do not make a right—meaning, in this case, the wrong that they did to you and the wrong you may do in retaliation. Find it in your heart, especially for a loved one, to show compassion when people are hurting. Many times the compassion you give will be returned to you, usually when you need it the most. Remember, we all make mistakes. Hate is defined as an intense hostility and aversion derived from fear, anger, or sense of injury, and extreme dislike or antipathy.

Hate has many root causes. It starts when a person feels they have been mistreated or wronged. Their emotions get the best of them, and that feeling can snowball into a disaster for them and others. The rock group Three Dog Night had a popular song titled "Easy to Be Hard." They pretty much ask the question, and I paraphrase, how can people be so heartless? In this book's first few chapters I discuss how there is a definite increase in everyone's selfishness in this century compared to the last one. That increased selfishness can reach levels of narcissism. Narcissists are extremely self-centered people who have an exaggerated sense of self-importance and narcissistic personality disorder. They also are people who are overly concerned with their physical appearance.

Interacting with people with narcissistic tendencies is difficult for everyone within their social group of friends, family, or sphere of influence. It's best that *anyone* who cares for a person showing signs of narcissism explain to them that their recent behavior has changed. Like alcoholism, the person with the problem has to understand they have the problem first, because they need professional therapy. The alcoholic is weak and trapped in their addiction and must first realize they have a problem. However, with narcissism it needs to be taken a step further. Alcoholism may not be caused by other people or society. There are sixteen things that may cause narcissists to hate: authority, vulnerability, commitment, criticism, loneliness, lack of admiration, lack of acknowledgement, insult, getting a "no" response, being wrong/apologizing, rejection, public humiliation, losing at anything, being ignored/abandoned, being challenged, or having rules changed. With narcissism the hatred manifests in selfish acts to retaliate with more hate toward the sender of the perceived first hateful act. When continual hateful acts occur and people become victimized, friends should help. In fairness, many acts of hatred occur innocently without premeditation. The results, however, still leave the victim with the feeling of receiving unfair treatment. It is what I call perception and reality, or PR: The perception of the narcissistic acts as acceptable and the reality of the fact that they are not. Friends, intermediators, or counselors should help when the hatred can lead to real harm and significant damage. Third-party intervention may convince the person that it is only perception not reality. If there are actual frequent acts of hatred, it is the third party's obligation to contact social services, thus preventing further mental or physical abuse to victims.

The friends and relatives of married couples hoped and prayed for the newlyweds at their weddings and hoped that their love for each other would last forever. It is unfortunate how the social pressures of the day can affect marriages. Things like your job, parenting, debt, and *all that stress that comes with it can be devastating.* Couples really should take more time to understand how those things may affect their marriage or relationship and take steps to prevent them. Our heritage, the one that guarantees religious beliefs, has helped many people cope with the pressures of our society. Most religions have clerics that understand what selfishness is. They understand what evil acts against humanity are and can provide comfort to help curb the pain caused by them.

One of this book's purposes was to highlight the dichotomy of the twentieth and the twenty-first centuries. It is really a double vision. There is a definite difference between the two centuries; I see it, and people my age see it too. It's about the people, technology and its use, and the stress being created. It *is* a culture change, self-inflicted by society. I have seen a recent example; it became apparent to me at the two high schools near my home. One school had a blue devil and the other a bee. The school's blue devil in the 1960s and '70s looked much like Duke University's blue devil logo, somewhat docile looking. Today that high school's logo looks like a devil with a hateful and mean face. The other high school has a bee logo. In the 1960s, the bee logo was a lovable flying honeybee. Today that honeybee is a fighting bee complete with stingers. You reap what you sow as parents and teachers. Which will you choose, *hate and stress or calmness and peace?* The most important thing that should be understood by the parents and children of school districts is that the districts were and are first and foremost institutions for academics and secondly for any other purpose. School fundamentally means a place to learn and also to become a beneficial and hopefully productive member of our society.

## DIVORCE

Your friends and relatives that went to your wedding did not go to it to see your marriage evaporate later. There is a lot of heat and evaporation with marriages, and those in attendance knew that. When they waved and saw you off on your voyage of matrimony they hoped and prayed for you. They were pleased to offer what they could. Many were married too and knew that every little bit given may help build your marriage.

Couples should discuss their reasons for divorce in a quiet, calm, constructive manner. They may find that their problems may be just PR: *perceptions instead of realities*. Perhaps it is rumored information by envious old friends that are now frenemies. *God damn social media*. Cell phone texting can lead to misunderstandings. It is because of the necessity to "get that little point out" quickly. However, many issues require a telephone call, or maybe even a face-to-face meeting to clearly get all the little facets of an issue out for understanding. It is important to remember that people come from many different backgrounds. Sometimes silly misunderstandings can be misconstrued and blown way out of proportion. Perhaps your partner has deep rooted behavior issues they are carrying with them. Please lay out your problems, differences, and difficulties and separately write them down and review them together. Maybe you can work them out.

In an earlier chapter I said that everything is a business and to be business-like. A marriage is a continuing construction project and, like a business operation, should be led by mature adults. The fact is businesses are either *growing or dying*. There is really very little wiggle room. Even if you choose the word *sustainability*, it takes *effort and expense for sustainability*. In business and in marriage, you only get out what is put into them. I'm not going to sugar coat it. All operations that run smoothly have a plan and a budget. The better the planning and budgeting, the better the results.

If you are contemplating a divorce from your marriage, I recommend that you list all of your options first. However, place reconciliation on the top of that list. Married couples, like a business, have put a lot of time, money, and effort into building it up. To tear it down may be more costly than building it up. I have a friend who considered divorcing his wife. His answer to finding the right option was, "It is cheaper to keep her." If you are having serious problems and reconciliation is out of the question, please either go to a marriage counselor or your religious organization to seek help. Those people are professionals and have a long list of satisfied customers.

On the subject of business and budgets in divorce, what is your attitude toward debt? Realistically, adults know, or should know, people cannot continue to raise their personal debt with no real, tangible way of paying it back. *Credit card debt is no different than having gambling debts.* Think of credit cards the same as dice. If you were to roll them, instead of coming up sevens, you keep coming up snake eyes. The only difference is that you are dealing with banks instead of the mob or the syndicate. The mob would beat the money out of you. Banks just stand in line for your bankruptcy case. My advice for young couples getting married is to have a budget and stick to it. *That includes zero debt!* You won't earn any awards from your friends for how you joined the crowd of America's "fashionable debtors" today. It is idiotic, and it causes your marriage an enormous amount of stress, and it impacts our country's debt as well.

There is nothing called "fashionable debtors." It was not meant as a joke. It really is a mental disease. It is called CBD: compulsive buying disorder. It is real and has caused marriages, families, and our country a tremendous amount of damage. We live in an over-advertised environment today and one that we did not have thirty years ago, before cable TV and the internet now linked to our little "sell"—I mean cell phones. CBD needs to be addressed before any "green deal." We have to fix the "red, white, and blue deal" first because this is a real problem for our economy. The items coming from overseas are not long-term investments like property, homes, and automobiles. Purchasing these low-equity, mostly perishable, judging by their quality, will not create higher-wage jobs here in America. That is where young people should be investing their money, especially when interest rates are very low. I discuss investment examples in chapter 17 on economics, chapter 18 on heath and pollution, and in the last chapter. Please invest some of your income in equitable ventures. It is an investment in your marriage and in America.

While you are mulling over the whys and why nots for divorce, do not forget about your children. They are almost always the forgotten ones in divorces. Divorce with children *is probably the first case for child abuse in America.* Why? Because when you consider a divorce you may be the first abusers. You inevitably are hurting them. Maybe not physically but emotionally. Children need stability, and divorce can cause instability. Just because divorce is on the rise statistically doesn't mean it is the right thing to do. I have a funny but sad way to describe divorce. If children are involved, there should be laws to make divorce illegal. That was only a sarcastic statement. Our children are our future and divorce may just be taking our nation a step backward. If you must divorce and have children, please know and understand that your close friends have you their prayers.

When I think about the triune of this chapter—love, hate and divorce—three songs ring in my ears. They were the inspiration for this chapter. They are "Respect," "You've Lost that Lovin' Feelin'," and "Open Arms." Each of the three reminds me of the phases that marriages may go through. The song "Respect" was sung by Aretha Franklin and written by Otis Redding. Aretha spells out to her lover *literally and letter-ly* how she deserves respect. When your actions toward each other are true, honest, and open, the respect for each becomes earned.

"You've Lost that Lovin' Feelin'" is performed by the Righteous Brothers and written by Barry Mann, Phil Spector, and Cynthia Weil. The song tells about the little things in a once loving relationship that has changed. It seems that it is always *the little things* (misunderstanding/misinterpretation) that can mushroom into big things. Communication is so important and always accentuates the positive. My wife is one of those people who always sees the positives in things. If you can maintain a positive attitude you will have done your part in removing any hate in your relationships.

The rock group Journey performs the song "Open Arms." Steve Perry sang it and cowrote it with Jonathan Cain. There is a genuine display of forgiveness in this song by the singer. [1]The poet Alexander Pope wrote, "To err is human; to forgive, divine." In the song "Open Arms," Steve Perry sings that he is hoping his lover will see what her love means to him, and therefore he must forgive her. That is why I hope couples can always forgive each other through their relationship together. Always hug each other like you did when you first fell in love. Go and hug each other now!

# 16.

# War and Pieces

Ask a soldier who spent time in a foxhole during a battle and they will say, "War is Hell!" I suppose it was a matter of destiny for our country, the United States of America, to begin in Hell. It began with a battle on the fields of Lexington and Concord against a tyrannical empire, Great Britain. The first significant event which enraged the colonists was the tea tax (Tea Act of 1773). Taxes have a way of doing that. The colonists called it "taxation without representation." We must understand the mindset of the colonists to revolt against the greedy administration of King George. Greedy, evil people or regimes, by their inhumane nature, cannot help themselves when feeding their selfishness. It was the same old story with Napoleon, the Spanish nobility, Germany's Kaiser, and Adolf Hitler, and it looks like Vladimir Putin's Russia and Communist China are the new evil empires.

Other than killing off many of the surface population through wars, what did these greedy regimes accomplish? I know one thing, each regime ended up losing! In Great Britain's case, it wasn't a World War I loss—they were on the winning side—but the unimaginable costs they paid due to the war itself. Those costs of the war caused the collapse of their empire. Other than the loss of lives, what significant accomplishments were made? What changes were made? The League of Nations? The United Nations? Those organizations haven't accomplished much other than housing diplomats and acting like they are doing something. Did they stop North Korea, Vietnam, Saddam Hussein, or Putin? What's next? Only President Reagan,

Pope John Paul II, and the Solidarity movement in Poland made a difference. They helped collapse an evil empire, the USSR. President Reagan said, "Peace through strength." I believe in proven effective methods. That method has been shown to work as a deterrent. There is nothing like having leverage at the negotiating table when the bargaining begins. Many people believe that the total withdrawal of United States troops, without securing a military base in Afghanistan, may have led to Russia's attack on Ukraine in 2022. Not putting American troops into strategic locations removes a large bargaining chip should diplomatic negotiations develop. Whether it is diplomacy or strong defenses, steps must be taken to prevent the direct loss of life, wars, the refugees they create, or any forced or paid migration of people. *All three of these are acts against humanity.*

It is important to fully comprehend the many hardships Americans suffered through, working hard to build this giant beacon for liberty, freedom, and democracy called America. It was *not* to prove to the world that the United States is or was the strongest, richest, or most compassionate country in the world. It was to prove to its own people— the pilgrims, pioneers, and immigrants—that it was a place for dreams and for families to grow should there be opportunities for them during *certain* times or circumstances. We did not ask for the wars we entered into. We were either attacked or drawn into them to prevent oppression and tyranny by evil people and the control they held over naïve or *unsuspecting* people. Similarly, it is what is happening to Ukraine and the Middle East today.

The United States through the years did not intend to start any of the military engagements they were involved with. They were sucked into them because of the effects that greedy nations or their leaders had, directly or indirectly. Some instances were a demarcation dispute (the Mexican War), or direct attacks (Pearl Harbor) and 9/11 (Afghanistan). I will admit, there was a real drive for manifest destiny in the United States, for a country from sea to sea, after the Louisiana Purchase from France.

Listed below are some of the death tolls from wars the United States has been engaged in.

- War of 1812 – 15,000 Americans and 6,000 British and Canadian soldiers died.
- Mexican War – 3,000 American soldiers died.
- Civil War – 618,222 soldiers died, 360,222 Union and 258,000 Confederate. (*Almost 250 Union soldiers died per day in the fight against slavery!*)
- Spanish-American War – 55,000 total soldiers died, 90 percent from diseases (malaria etc.).
- World War I – 10 million military personnel and 5 million civilians died.
- World War II – 20 million military personnel and 40 million civilians died.
- Vietnam War – 47,434 American soldiers and 9,500 non-military personnel died.
- Mideast/Afghanistan Conflicts – 7,054 American military personnel died.

Some of Hollywood's most recent war movies are very graphic when it comes to the human "pieces." The movie *Pearl* is about the Japanese Empire's attack on the United States at Pearl Harbor. *Pearl* was about the barbaric and brutal surprise attack on a naïve, neutral nation. The movie made you feel as though you were at that attack on Pearl Harbor in Hawaii. The viewer saw our soldiers being blown to pieces, drowning, or burning in a pool of fire. Yes, war is hell.

In the movie *Saving Private Ryan*, the scenes from Omaha Beach in Normandy, France, were even more graphic. You saw soldiers being ripped to shreds by German gunners that were stationed high atop the landing beach area. The world needed a western front to turn the tide of war, and the United States provided it. Thousands of American soldiers died at Normandy (125,847). Many are still lying there at the St. Laurent Cemetery in Colleville-sur-Mer, France. Yes, war is hell!

Our Memorial Day, a federal holiday, almost doesn't feel like a holiday at all. When we remember the veterans, like my dad, it reminds me of the price our nation paid for saving the freedoms and liberties we enjoy every day. For some reason, as after World War I, "the war to end all wars," we keep letting our guard down. We enjoy the peace in the world but forget how some humans and nations are hell bent on power and greed. They are lurking in the shadows, weeds, or trees like opportunist predators. These are some of the worst evildoers. Why are most of the world's journalists not working to uncover these potential threatening nations in their stories? It makes one wonder. Other than a press release, people need to be reminded of the selfishness of real evil, not TV shows about fake things like zombies. It is about the bad things people do to other people. I hope the news media can save the "feel good" stories when all of the bad actions of the day are cleaned up first. That can only happen when the *good people* of a nation really care about common, everyday people, the ones just trying to make a living.

Another Memorial Day thought I have is about President Abraham Lincoln. He sat in the hottest seat ever in the White House. Many of his words are carved in granite, in our history, and in our memories. In the Gettysburg Address which he wrote he said, "We here highly resolve that these dead shall not have died in vain, that this nation, under God, shall have a new birth of freedom, and that government of the people, by the people, for the people, *shall not perish from the earth*." Another of his famous statements was, "A house divided against itself cannot stand."

For this chapter, my inspiration came from the song "What's Going On." It was written by Marvin Gaye, Renaldo Benson, and Al Cleveland, and performed by Marvin Gaye. The song tells about how there are too many mothers crying because their sons (or daughters) they raised are dying in wars. I believe sometimes mothers are a little too silent about their outward emotions for their adult children. They do not want those young adults to carry the burden of their worries about them as they may be called off to war to defend our nation.

There is one thing that I am glad did not happen when discussing the two aforementioned movies, *Pearl* and *Saving Private Ryan*. It is that the mothers of those brave soldiers were long dead and did not have to relive the horror of thinking that their young adults died in that frightening fashion. It was by God's grace that those parents passed away without having to see how their brave young soldiers were shredded to pieces or burned to save nations from powerful, aggressive monsters that feed off of naïve, freedom-loving people. I do believe that for us to thwart off any evil nations in our world we must understand that the best defense begins with a good offense. President Ronald Reagan was right when he said, "Peace through strength."

# 17.

# Government, Economics, Politics, and Our Defense

This chapter has four parts that are interwoven. They are Economics, Politics, Our Defense, and most importantly, Government. Government is the glue that can manage them and create a lean, mean working machine—or take it down. What makes a working democracy great is that it inherently is a participative style of government. There has not been a better participative style of government than what we have been blessed with. That is what democracy is all about. It has been working fairly well in the United States of America for nearly 250 years. (It has been the envy of the world for those who strive for their citizenry to have participative government, and condemned by authoritarians). It is for that reason this chapter is dedicated to reminding families and friends to be continuously aware that authoritarian governments or groupings of our own citizenry may work to take our democracy (choices) away from us.

Believe it or not, our country has adversaries. We have seen it in the past and the present. There have been military forces (Britain, Spain, Japan), economic competitors (Soviet Union), and religious zealots (9/11, case in point). Those adversaries are all for ending our democracy. The educated know and understand that *envy and egos are dangerous things.* Many years ago, I used to tell my friends that government and economics should be as separate as church and state, as stated in our Constitution. It was that way before our entry into both World Wars. President Teddy Roosevelt and others around the beginning of the twentieth century realized the damage that the ultra-rich elitists can cause to a free-market economy. The industrial giants then monopolized the marketplaces and removed any attempt to compete in those markets. Believe it or not, Teddy Roosevelt, a Republican, and his followers were called "progressives" in their day. That word has a whole different meaning today, maybe even "regressive." The Teddy Roosevelt progressives back then worked to ensure that regulations were in place to protect the general public in the United States from powerful controlling entities. After World War II, when the United States became the defender of freedom and democracy throughout the world, the need to have a large standing military required our government to be in the military business. The Soviet Union was the evil empire then, forcibly pushing their communist manifesto and authoritarian government throughout the world, Cuba being an example. This led to more international security, *but at a cost*. We will cover the economics part of government in more detail later in this chapter.

When discussing government, I tell my friends that a government, like any church, is only as good as its pastor. Either the congregation is active and smiling, or they are leaving on their own or because of a pandemic, for instance. For churches, leadership is of the utmost importance, and how they manage their church is essential. I learned an important lesson about organizations from a comedy movie I once saw. An auto parts manufacturer was explaining his business's survival on its continual growth. From his line I began to understand that every organization is a business. Not in the sense of a profiteering enterprise, but business-like in functioning. The big box stores, your electric company, your city, the Red Cross, the Salvation Army, your public library, schools and colleges, communist China, and even your family are all businesses. Every organization, even a single volunteer giving their time and talent in any attempted venture, is a business. Everything has people in its operation, and they all must (or should) work together to make it successful and hopefully useful for humanity. Why should anyone waste an education or their experience on something called "busy work." Firefighters and military personnel may seem static at times; however, their duties are to be prepared to respond to life's unforeseen emergencies. Yes, everything, *especially governments, are businesses.*

When I use the word *organization*, I means any group of people working together for a purpose. When any business starts, the organizers know that profits or donations are necessary to satisfy at least the bank's requirements to keep the organization solvent. However, they also must have insight into what their organization may look like in the future, when it becomes more than just a profit or service enterprise and takes on the responsibility of being perhaps the fundamental resource for the livelihood of everyone in that organization. I have worked in both the private sector and the public sector all my life. I found it amazing how some organizations (which means people) can thrive and grow, and others die. Yes, the overall economic climate can affect them, but most of the time it is just the decisions being made by the branch of the organization called "the management" that can make or break the business. The good organizations understand that they need feedback from everyone in the organization. All employees in the organization should be stakeholders and in essence part of the management. Positions in organizations have different duties and responsibilities. However, like a chain, it is only as strong as its weakest link. Egos should be left outside the door, because many times they are selfish notions and a "turnoff." The rank and file in time figure out what the business is about and the need for interdependence among everyone. These people understand how important it is to be enabled to provide operational feedback of information so good decisions can be made by management. That coincidentally is also how the good democratic governments work. Everyone must have good verifiable information from which to make decisions, and many truthful pipelines to receive it.

## GOVERNMENT

I have a simple question for you. Do you want to be a dog wagging its tail, or have the tail wag *you* (the dog)? When we use words to describe our democracy, we say our government is "of the people, by the people, and for the people." In a typical democracy, such as ours, the citizens must be active participants. You, the voter, are the dog, and Congress, the representatives that you elected, are the tail. That is how our democracy and a republic were designed to work. The tail wagging the dog is called communist socialism, imperialism, and the like. A dictionary states that government is : 1) the act of governing, 2) process of governing, 3) the office, authority or function of governing, and 4) can be described as a group of people who control and make decisions for a country, state, and local places. It also is the system for countries, states, and other places to be controlled.

Psychologists have studied human fundamental needs over the last one hundred years (figure 17A shows Abraham Maslow's hierarchy of needs). Our human basic needs are listed at the bottom of the pyramid. These needs must be met by individuals themselves, for the bare necessities of life, or entrusted to another institution: government. Once basic needs are met, one can start to move upward toward less important needs, or their wants. That is why a democratic form of government offers liberties and freedom of thought for action. Figure 17-B illustrates many of the world's common forms of government. Democratic forms of government provide a person the best opportunity to achieve self-direction and incentives. That system inherently fosters values and opinions. However, democracies are fragile. I repeat: *Democracies are fragile.* That point about democracies must be understood, *respected, and protected.*

There are external countries and internal interest groups that are either envious of our democracy or are misled to believe it causes strife. However, there are times where poor leadership in governments can cause strife. An economy may cause strife, but not democracy itself. Communism, for instance, is a governmental group in total control of its people. It purposely limits a person from any self-direction. It places them in a ready-made pool of the controlling group's design and purpose. An average person ("anonymous person" is better for this example) is excluded from participating in any planning or modification in that organization unless chosen by that party. The beneficiary of that system is the group that maintains and controls it, especially the country's money. The key word is *control*. Either you are "in with the in crowd, or out with the out crowd." So much for any participation in that style. The only incentive in that system is to show the controlling group that *you*, the anonymous one, the controlled one, have been a loyal "minion" and deserve to be with the in crowd. A person has a better chance of winning the lottery than being in a participative position in communist socialism. Quite simply put, a baby born in a democracy has an opportunity for self-direction and participation, but a baby born into communist socialism already has their life planned for them by a small group for that *group's own benefit*.

In our democracy Congress controls our money, but through democracy, we are supposed to control Congress. That is why it is so important for every American to choose their representatives very carefully. Do the representatives solicit the thoughts and opinions of their voting base, or do they represent only their personal agenda, political donors' needs, or worse, a closed-minded ideology? I have mentioned Congress often. However, our country is a conglomeration of states; therefore, many times it is just as important, maybe even more important, to have governors who have their state's citizens' best interest at heart instead of any party line's business objectives. Governors are voted into office to manage their state, but in doing so they are to respect your opinions, run the state as successful, debt-free operations, and keep their citizenry safe. They must work to gather the majority of their citizens' needs, or they have misled or disenfranchised them. They must honor their oath of office before entering the office.

Make no mistake, when you pay your hard-earned tax money to governments, you entrust them to run the government effectively and efficiently. It is incumbent on any successful organization to manage its station and make its operations transparent to its external and internal customers. By internal customers I mean every person in that organization. In government, that is its legal citizenry. If you want the team all working in the same direction, they need to see the group's direction every day. Everyone should see their value in the organization, their need for interdependence, and their progress through whatever measurement tools are available. For a country, their gross national product or gross national income are examples. States are supposed to show growth not debt, or they are only a burden to the overall growth of the nation. The transparency part is that their activities are producing beneficial products or services that are not harmful to anyone. All mistakes must be corrected and openly admitted. Regulations are the laws enacted for those assurances. The activities are not the ends to the means but only the means to a rewarding life. Not just for an individual, but for everyone. Our democracy was not created for any political group to govern our country. It is our responsibility to have assurances that our country is being managed fairly, effectively, and efficiently.

Recreational activities for everyone in the organization, or country, are as important as the positions everyone holds. I discussed this in chapter 6, "Distractions to Your Goals." Since a government is the composition of its citizenry, a government's health and self-preservation are dependent on the mental and physical health of its people. For the health of a fragile democratic system, it is important that all political candidates respect its fragility, represent their constituents, and assure that its fundamental principles are not compromised.

There have been hundreds of books written about management styles. From Frank and Lillian Gilbreth's books on efficiency, to Peter

Drucker's *Management by Objectives* and W. Edwards Deming's teaching of *Total Quality Management.* I believe in the seven M's of management. They are manpower, material, machinery, money, methods, m-powerment (empowerment), and magic (innovation, integrity, and intangibles). The methods of management are the important ones. *Proven effective methods* should be the choices. Those methods usually produce positive outcomes. The management must remain active and not be passive. Problems occur in all organizations and, if not responded to, only fester and get worse. The organization's participants expect its leadership to resolve its problems. They expect its leadership to do so, or they lose faith in their leadership. Make no mistake, *all governments are businesses.* A case in point is the communist Soviet Union, the USSR. That is a story about how a country can begin with a revolution, and how it can die. I am sure the communist Chinese have thought about the USSR often and believe they have figured that one out.

In 1973, while attending college, I was required a write a research paper for my English 102 course. I choose the topic "Trade Unions are as Democratic as the Soviet Union." I did all the required research and needed to prove my statement and theory. The point was that the communist Soviet Union rated a zero on the democratic-principle scale, because it was a totalitarian form of government. I provided examples of my own trade union experiences. I had two at the time, and other examples from my research. I explained that most trade unions have no internal parties. They are a one-party system, which limits the union's control on ideas and growth. Also, many do not have a system of checks and balances and leave their treasuries open to the potential of theft. I explained that one trade union, the International Typographical Union, had a two-party system. In that system, both parties had a basic platform. One party was the founding party. Their platform was to negotiate its workers' contract with its employers. The other, the newer party's platform, was the more aggressive one. They took a position to strike against their employers. The research paper required a conclusion. I concluded that the two-party system was more democratic, more participative, and therefore the better choice. We have a two-party system in our government. For our sake, let us make sure a one-party system can never occur. If it does, the controlling group would most likely dissolve our democracy, because it would not benefit them (the one controlling party).

Historically, the pharaohs of Egypt, the Roman Empire, the dynasties of China, Great Britain's "ruling the waves," and the communist Soviet Union all had governments that were established for some purpose. Some succeeded and others failed. The United States has always supported the principle to learn about our history, world history, and the need to be a freethinking country. Some misled Americans may forget that the freethinking education they enjoy was achieved by ideals and sacrifices made to insure our democracy. The misled too quickly forget there was a price to pay for having the freedom for that education. A respect for those who sacrificed themselves for those principles requires a dedication to defend our nation and its democratic DNA. If we are to have a sustainable government *of the people, by the people, and for the people*, all of the people are responsible to take up the burden of the costs for those liberties and have the duty to preserve them. Freedom is not free. Thomas Jefferson said you have the right to life, liberty, and pursuit of happiness. Hopefully your neighbor is not some anarchist with an agenda to derail your life's vision, nor the one Thomas Jefferson had in his mind for your pursuit of happiness. Also remember the tax issue. Your income is your income unless you decide to give it away for higher taxes and bigger government. It is your choice. The income you make can build your security blanket and is leverage to help keep our liberties and freedom. Keep America lean and mean. Do not let your elected representatives think that government is only a process or a game and not a business. Simply put, higher taxes take your liberties and freedoms away from you. About 90 percent of my college professors in government, social studies, and economics classes stated,

"Smaller government is better government." They must have understood the faults of some people, so choose your representatives carefully.

## ECONOMICS

One of our more famous American presidents was Calvin Coolidge. He had some famous words for a group of Americans during one of his speeches. He said, "After all, the chief business of the American people is business. They are profoundly concerned with producing, buying, selling, investing, and prospering in the world." He gave that speech during an address to the American Society of Newspaper Editors in Washington, DC, on January 17, 1925. In that address he cautioned those working in the newspaper business about the role of the press, and warned them about the evils of propaganda. That was almost a hundred years ago. From these words we should take away those two important points. Can our mass media today, other than constantly bombarding us with advertising, emphasize the importance of displaying a businesslike attitude? The rest of the world is watching us. On the propaganda point, I would hope that the media would once again just report all news and not sensationalize it for any political purposes.

I often emphasize the importance of the fact that governments are businesses too, or, better stated, must be businesslike. One of my reasons is that a poorly run government can go into what is called default, when an entity is unable to pay its debts. This happened on December 15, 1978, to my childhood city, Cleveland, Ohio. It took almost two years for the city to become solvent again. Cleveland became the first major city in the United States to default on its debts. It was a national embarrassment. Yes, governments are businesses.

I previously mentioned that a comedy movie inspired me to realize that businesses must either grow or die. That is so true, and it is mostly about how they are organized. In chapter 9 on religion, we discussed the two simple elements of good and evil. In economics, the simple elements are supply and demand. In the section on government, we discussed how people have basic needs for their survival (see figure 17-A). They are food, clothing, and shelter. Fortunately, most Americans today have a multitude of products to meet those basic needs. When their basic needs are met, people begin to climb up Maslow's triangle of hierarchy and begin their quest to acquire their "wants." These will hopefully help produce a better YOU. In turn, you will not only achieve your personal goals, but as a member of society you will hopefully produce better products and services and improve your family's well-being. This is your personal economic growth. In your personal sense this is called microeconomics. It affects your household and is part of the mechanism that economists use to judge and gauge resources for producing products and services that you have purchased in the marketplace. When combining the economics across the field of others in marketplaces it is called macroeconomics.

Money is the medium of exchange based on some agreed-upon standard of value. For years countries have used the metals silver and gold or jewels as that standard. Assets are the goods you have acquired for either your basic needs or your improvement. Having assets, usually the products or goods in your household, will increase economic growth. For a country, it's collectively the overall growth. The assets have a value, and maintaining that value is a stabilizing factor for a country's economy. The prices for those goods and services are set by the quantity of supply and the amount of demand. The more the supply, the price typically can go down. The more demand, the price goes up. With the advent of computers, interpreting data relative to supply and demand has helped individuals and all markets and industries in the world. Computers forecast production, which stabilizes pricing and eliminates the waste of over-producing. In most countries businesses are taxed on their produced products and their unsold inventory.

A major question for everyone trying to achieve economic growth is: Do the assets you have acquired exceed the amount of money you owe (debt)? Subtracting the amount of debt from the assets equates to equity. For homeowners, the amount of equity you invest in your home or business increases your financial security or its bottom-line value. Most people understand that owning property and paying lower property taxes makes it a worthwhile investment. Automobile purchases can be a good or a bad investment. Achieving reliable low-cost transportation for commuting to your employment is a positive thing. Automobile dealers can make a profit when buying and selling automobiles. However, purchasing an automobile and seeing it rapidly decrease in value in its first two years could make it a bad investment. Products that are considered convenience or pacifying items can be bad investments, like cable TV, gambling, gaming, and alcohol. Their value is temporary and decreases your income. The money that you can save is an asset. The point is, if everyone in a marketplace experiences economic growth, it increases the country's total economic growth. Countries are marketplaces. Your personal debt has a negative effect on the overall value of your equity. If everyone has a higher debt against their assets, the value of their country's equity can have a stifling effect on a country's economic growth. It is life's simple balance sheet of income and expenses. You are the manager of your income and your expenses, and that requires a budget.

Since the 1700s, to deal with debt, countries have established their own central banks. These banks keep cash on hand to meet any unexpected demand for withdrawals. Since the late 1990s, and due to disasters like the Great Depression, the World Bank has functioned in that capacity. However, each country is still responsible to limit its debt. Debt is unfavorable because it compromises a country's rating value for banks to lend money. Basically, higher debt causes a country to be a bad investment. Being able to have economic growth and not having debt is important because lenders charge interest on any debt, and debt limits growth.

A trade deficit occurs when your country or its citizenry buys more products or services than it sells. These products and services all have monetary values. Economists argue that balance of trade does not have any bearing on economic impact for a country. However, if you look at balance of trade in a microeconomic sense, where you are purchasing more than you are producing, the value of your assets decreases because of your inability to acquire loans to achieve a manageable balance. You now have a lesser value than your trading partner.

Here is a list of some dictionary definitions for economic terms:

- National debt is the amount of money that a government owes to companies and countries.
- A trade deficit occurs when a country buys more from foreign countries than it sells to them.
- Balance of trade is the difference in value between a country's imports and exports in time.
- Inflation is a steady rise in prices attributed to increasing the volume of money and credit for the goods and services available.
- Gross national product (GNP) is the total value of goods produced and services provided by a country for one year. It is equal to the gross domestic product plus the net income from foreign investments.
- Gross national income (GNI) is the total domestic and foreign output claimed by residents of a country, consisting of gross domestic product, plus factor incomes earned by foreign residents, minus income earned in the domestic economy by nonresidents.

I like the system of using the GNP over the GNI, which is now used. The GNP is true income as income because the end result is a product that has a tangible value. However, credit card lending institutions, not necessarily home mortgage lenders, are making up to 25 percent interest on your purchases. Our nation's penchant for buying to feed our vanity only helps the bigger corporations and foreign traders (like communist China) to increase their income while your income is lowered by the outrageously high interest rates. We must remember, Communist China is an economic trading partner but also a trading adversary. The GNP reflects the products that we produce, the assets, and those are our valued products, which typically, in the manufacturing sense, also produce higher-paying jobs.

Another fundamental of economics besides supply and demand is the basic result of a productive economic system: COMPETITION. Competition in a marketplace is essential to place "real" values on assets, and helps establish its pricing. Competition leads to innovations and better ways "to build better mouse traps" as they say. It causes organizations to continually review their products or services to adjust their costs, improve them, and make them more profitable for the organization. Our country's freedom to choose our vocations produces the motivation in people to learn more about those fields of endeavor. This is the challenge for our education system. Elementary education should begin to foster that thought and creativity for our children. At one time programs like Junior Achievement were introduced to our high schoolers.

Let us have some fun playing some games to use as an example of how microeconomics effects macroeconomics. That is how personal households can affect global interests. Two popular board games will be used as an example. I love to play board games. There is no better way to engage a family than playing board games. These games have it all over those expensive electronic games that mostly engage children individually rather than socially. The electronic pads will be obsolete soon enough and will be another piece of junk in the waste can. We already have too many concerns about the increase in the world's garbage as pollution. I will discuss that subject in chapter 18, "Our Health, Food, Environment, and Pollution."

The two games I enjoyed playing the most were the game of Life and Monopoly. Having your country's debt or trade imbalance grow is much like being a player in one of those games. For our example, imagine eight people in a room with two tables. They have four people at one table playing the game of Life and four at the other table playing Monopoly. The two bankers from each group distribute the play money among the players in each group before the two games begin. In the game of Life, the players are having children and trying to raise them in a positive environment, beginning with good schools in hopes of them gaining useful employment. In the Monopoly game, the players know one thing. *It is a last-person-standing and winner-take-all game.* While both games are going on, the bankers from both games agreed to use their money interchangeably to buy items from each other's games, much like a trade agreement. At one point, a player from the game of Life wants and purchases Chance and Community Chest cards from the Monopoly game. That player's reasoning was simply to own the cards. In actuality, Chance and Community Chest cards only function as "operational pieces" in the game of Monopoly. They have very little value compared to the real estate, industry, or utility cards played in the Monopoly game. The card sales transaction between the games resulted in one of the game of Life players having less cash on hand. Although it is the individual player's loss, relative to microeconomics, it lowered the amount of available cash and the overall equity and buying power of their group's game. However, the Monopoly game and its players acquired more cash on hand (equity) and increased the value and amount of money that each player could play with (growth).

There are lessons learned from playing the above economic games. Equity increases and decreases are examples of economic growth and failures. Our world's games of life (families) and monopolies (selfish actualization) have real meanings. In those games, for one group it was for everyone to play and compete to see how the families could grow and benefit. However, for the other group, the winner-take-all one, it was purely a lesson on who gets to control the board with their winnings. A lesson learned from these games is to know the mission of your trading partners. Another lesson is that the world of economics *is a tough business*; therefore, be prepared.

Over one hundred years ago, the United States had the same problem with our economy, just like the examples given in our board games. Back then it was powerful business entities like Standard Oil and our nation's largest railroads. Those companies and the industries they represented became monopolies and limited competition. Their actions controlled the production of certain supplies in key markets and allowed them to set prices at unrealistic values. President Teddy Roosevelt was a defender for more competition in the marketplaces and helped initiate laws to curb controlling marketplace activities. Today, we are suffering with many of those same problems. Large powerful groups are controlling various marketplaces and affecting everyone's buying power. We once again let the term *free enterprise* be mistaken for *fair enterprise*. Only a system that has limits and regulations can achieve fairness and economic growth for everyone. In our country, the first major regulations were the antitrust laws enacted during President Teddy Roosevelt's time. Those regulations provided for a fair system of economics and put controls in marketplaces that produce goods and services. There is a price to pay for those regulations by government, but those regulations protect its citizens. The necessary regulations strengthen the integrity of the economic system, build opportunities, and promote a fair economic structure.

In America, over the past thirty years since the collapse of the Soviet Union, we have been playing our "game of life" with the future of our children (much like the players played the game above). I remember discussing this economic philosophy with a supervisor in our firm in the mid-1990s. He told me that the United States is transitioning from a manufacturing-base nation to a service one. He had just received his master's degree in business management. I told him that it would be foolish to transform to a service nation because it would limit the creation of tangible goods or assets (values) and cause increases in services (expenses). His answer was, "Well, that's the direction we are heading." He was right. For the last thirty years we have stopped our manufacturing and increased our services. What did we tangibly do to deserve an increase in our appetite for services? Did we work smarter or harder? The answer is: We did not work smarter. Our banking system got into the plastic money credit card business, and we all increased our debt. The only country that worked harder through this was Communist China because they increased their manufacturing capabilities to sell us cheaper, poor—quality goods with little value. This is a free global market, but not a fair global market, and has caused a debt problem. Economically, this is where we are at today. A historical and statistical fact is that the manufacturing jobs of our country's past created more valuable assets and provided higher-paying jobs in those industries. Why did they? Simply because those people back then worked harder and sweated more in those jobs, like our higher-paying construction jobs today. Sitting at a computer doing something called work does not compare to the amount of labor expended in the manufacturing industries. Manufacturing industries and their capabilities also assure our nation's ability to rapidly produce military equipment for our defense purposes *if and when needed.* We will touch further on our defense later in this chapter.

We should all work hard every day to be independent thinkers. I believe in the free and fair enterprise system, with the opportunities it brings. Our history has shown that limits and regulations to the free enterprise system must be continual, and the present ones need to be modified. Unfortunately, in the middle of all this business of economics is our system of defense. Historically, it was our great manufacturing ability that led us to victories in both world wars. Without a manufacturing base, how are we to produce the necessary tools for our defense? Herein lies our problem. From the little manufacturing done in America I believe you can see how defenseless we are. We must fix this security problem! We must return to manufacturing our own products of high quality that have value. Well-made equipment is essential for our defense. This equipment *must not fail* as often as the poorly made products produced overseas.

Reading the many philosophies about economic growth, that is from a total hands-off approach (Laissez-faire) to total control of it (Communism) makes economics appear to be field of no hardcore answers. Many governments have tried what is called trickle-down (from businesses downward) to supply-side (trickle-up) induced with special interest political economics. By my observations either can work or not work given an array of circumstances the economy is presently in. For instance what is the strength of the currency and the citizen's attitudes. I am avid gardener, and I see economic growth much like plant growth. I had an opportunity to teach 6th-graders in plant photosynthesis. I explained to them that three basic components are necessary for plant growth. They are sunlight (energy), good soil, and water. However, good maintenance by motivated believers (the gardeners) is essential for a good results, otherwise the plants would die. In economics those similar basic elements are needed. They are the energy, needed to produce ANYTHING, stable tangible resources, currency backed by real assets like gold, and the continued trickling of monetary funds by speculating investors. I have the fortune of witnessing economic growth in the USA economy between 2016-2019. It wasn't trickle-down or supply-side. It was accomplished by an infusion of the money from its own citizens, with tax refunds acting like fertilizers to plants, which generated the economic growth. I call that process "lateral nurturing economics" accomplished by a believing faithful citizenry. That economy began to whither on the vine by an attack from by invading virus from an economic competitor.

## POLITICS

In an earlier chapter I mentioned one of my favorite high school mentors, my social studies teacher, Fred Schuld. He would often read excerpts from a periodical that had a section titled "How the World Views Us" (the United States). I always think about that when I see the actions or inactions of our government when the world requires our intervention. I have been observing an attitude by many Americans that much of world events either do not matter to them or they feel it is out of their hands. If the world is watching the United States as a supposed example of democracy and leadership in our world, I believe we better start changing that oblivious attitude. Beginning with our politicians, that attitude better change, or the United States will be standing in the same breadlines as the rest of the third-world nations.

Politics for me started when I was seven years old. This coincided with the 1960 presidential election and the televised debates. Even back then, our black-and-white television alone showed how TV may influence its viewers' perception of candidates. For example, one TV debate showed how a young energetic JFK looked compared to Richard Nixon, with his five-o'clock shadow on his stubbly, unshaven face. I remember asking my mother what the debates were about. The debates were interrupting my favorite TV programs like the *Mickey Mouse Club*, *Lassie*, or the *Lone Ranger*. My mother explained that the candidates were running for offices *to represent us* in our government. I asked her for whom she was voting. With that she took a promotional flyer from the mail, with a photograph of a local politician running for office. She bent the card longways until the short corners matched, then pushed the center of the fold inward, flapping the short sides up and down like a chattering mouth. That ended my mom's lesson to me. She really did have a sense of humor.

As a stay-at-home mom at that time, and as my earliest mentor, the politics of the day may not have mattered much to her. She thought politicians were a bunch of do-gooders trying to get into office to avoid real work. After those sixty years since her lessons, we still have that problem. However, as my mom explained to me, they were candidates running for office *to represent us*. Our school textbooks tell us how our elected officials are supposed to represent us, just as my mom told me in 1960. However, once mixing the "party power of politics" distractions into what was supposed to be about their customers, the voters, *we the people,* the main purpose of their positions gets lost. Incidentally, after being a stay-at-home mom, my mother later entered the workforce, eventually became a union steward, and usually voted for Democratic candidates. However, she did vote for President Nixon in 1972, like almost everyone in our country did. He eventually learned to shave more.

I can remember the 2016 election and debates. While I worked in the public sector, the residents in their community would ask me my choice of candidates. I would explain to them as a government employee that it was unethical for me to discuss my choices specifically. Many of them told me they were voting for Donald Trump. The people of the State of Ohio supported him then, as they also did in 2020. I asked them in 2016 why they were supporting Donald Trump. They told me they were tired of party politics and the status quo in Washington, DC. It appeared to them that all the legislators were only interested in their personal interests and not ours. They said that an outsider to party politics was needed to get them, the legislators, to get the hint. I had people, mostly women, tell me they were voting for Hilary Clinton. Many of them said that Donald Trump was a millionaire, therefore they could not fundamentally vote for him. I did explain to them, though, that not being in politics, Donald Trump assuredly made his money on his time clock or his company's time. I mentioned that point purposely to plant that cue, because I did know that many politicians ended up much wealthier while working on *my* tax-paid time. Ethics, however, is lost in today's win-at-any-cost ideology, has lost its goodness for that practice.

Anyway, that typically was the extent of my political discussions with them. Their comments implied that there is a pot of gold at the end of the rainbow in Washington, DC. It is there for politicians to lasso some of it and to dole it out to their backers and special interest groups. I suppose that can happen. That was the same theme in that old classic movie, *Mr. Smith Goes to Washington*, wherein Jimmy Stewart (of *It's a Wonderful Life* fame) plays a newly elected junior senator and gets mistakenly linked to a real-estate construction scam. However, the scam was actually being done by his state's senior senator and not him.

*¹Politics* is described in a dictionary as: 1 a: the art or science of government, b: the art or science concerned with guiding or influencing governmental policy, c: the art or science concerned with winning and holding control over a government. 2: political action, practices, or policies, 3 a: political affairs or business ; competition between competing interest groups. ²A politician is described as: b: a person primarily interested in political offices from selfish or other narrow usu. short-run interests. From these definitions it is easy to see how an inducement to wrong by improper or unlawful means (such as bribery) can occur. Most importantly though, they are the political opinions or sympathies of a person.

After researching what politics are I find it a concern and even frightening. There is not one description above about the role of the politician to *represent their constituents*. That is where we are today in American politics. Why are we not taking charge and control of important defining roles in our society? Not just the politicians, but what about parenting? We are, according to our Constitution, to be in charge of this nation and our children, not the government. Our major adversaries in the world would like nothing better than to have us become an overweight, selfish, and lazy nation. Why? Because it would mean they won! As mentioned in our section on government, do you want to be the dog wagging its tail or the tail wagging the dog? Remember in chapter 3, "Your Character, Our Country, and Our Culture" when we discussed the word *culture*. Do you want *our* culture to be the reactive definition to describe the results of our actions as described in chapter 3? Or would you rather have our politicians work to shape our government like a cultured pearl, where we create a taste in fine arts, humanities, and broad aspects of science. Also, please add the word *ethics* to that list.

In this twenty-first century, more than ever in our history, we are distracted by our vanity. Due to those distractions, we are enabling a bunch of politicians to run amok with our tax money. It is happening on the local, state, and especially on the national level. Today's Congress, although having a variety of vocational backgrounds, do *not* have the same backgrounds as your average American neighborhood. Our politicians are rising from their local political positions by winning their election campaigns. Their successes, however, are due to their supporters' influence, public-speaking abilities, and knowledge of politics itself. Do not forget the incentive of political networking that awaits them as they climb up that ladder to the top, and the pot of gold.

We should elect representatives who understand from their experiences the reality of what Americans feel and experience every day. The young politicians are great at telling people what they think you want to hear. However, because of their youth, most have not experienced the hardships many Americans face firsthand. They retrieve feedback about your interests from two-dimensional sources like smartphones, big-screen TVs, or classroom lectures. There is the important third-dimension depth in value judgements not able to be seen on LCD screens. They do not see the actual feelings of their constituents and their physical experiences. They fail to understand the jobs that we do, or the feelings when negative actions hurt people (harassments, layoffs, suspensions, bankruptcy, home repossessing, or being fired). Two-dimensional screens do not transmit the "quality" of physical experiences. The Dr. Phils and Ozes try to explain these things, but you must live with them. These two great TV personalities are the first ones to tell you that fact about needing real experiences. As far as the doctors and lawyers go, there are some great ones that represent us. *They get it.*

I believe all elected legislators should sign a written copy of the oaths that they pledged when they entered into their elected positions. Included should be a copy of the US citizenship oath. They should repeat it from those documents to a standing judge, verbatim, detailing the terms of the agreement. If they do not fulfill the terms of the agreement, there should be mechanisms in place to relieve them of their duties. It should not matter what political position is held; if they are representing their political party's agenda over the safety and needs of their constituents, they should be replaced. I often hear about proposals to limit the terms for our congressional legislators. That could help with many of the political problems we face. All elected officials must be held accountable for their actions or inactions in their positions as our representatives. The voting public should be allowed by petition to remove any representatives who are negligent in the performance of their duties, especially if they mismanage the financials.

In earlier chapters we stated that you only get out of anything in life what you put into it. If you sense a problem in our government, you need to open your eyes more often and ask yourself if your representatives are working for you or themselves. The fundamental principle of this great democracy of ours was for you to be the controlling participant of our government. Like the owners of a business. I have been saying, everything is a business, and for sure the government is a business. Like successful sole proprietorships, elected representatives should be the first ones to open their office doors in the morning, turning on the lights, etc., and be the last ones to leave. The good entrepreneurs lead by example because many times their good names are on their businesses. In our various governments' cases, our good name is on the front of our cities, states, and country. If we are delegating responsibilities of our ownership of our government to representatives, our employees in this case, paid by our tax money, we need to get the best ones to do that. I have an important question. Should we hire a representative, a worker, who does not like our company, our leadership, and our ideals? Let us take the time for our business's life's sake, for our country's life's sake, to reevaluate our staff and remind them who they are working for. If they do not get it, show them the door. Historically, countries have called that defenestration. It is not a revolution, it is just a rethinking for the reason why our country's business, our democracy, sometimes loses its focus and direction and gets out of control.

We sometimes forget how little cues in our day may affect our thinking. Things such as a smiling little emoji on a text for instance. Probably one of the most important cues that has changed in our nation's political analysis has been how our major networks changed the colors representing each political party on election maps. For forty-five years, since the advent of color television, Republican states were represented with the color blue, and Democratic states with red. This changed about fifteen years ago because one political candidate supposedly mistakenly said that red represented Republican states. Since then, all the major news networks ran with it. That candidate and those TV networks forgot the reason that networks chose the color blue for Republican states. The reason was (and it should be flipped back to that former practice) because of Abraham Lincoln. He was the first Republican president, and the leader of the armed forces that fought to abolish slavery in America. His army wore blue hats and uniforms. Therefore, out of respect for those who died in that cause, they chose the color blue to represent Abraham Lincoln's army.

By the actions of radical left socialists during the pandemic years of 2020 and 2021, you remember the summer of love for Democratic governors. It only seems logical for the Democratic Party to return to their former color of red for election mapping. My reasoning is that those states, and unfortunately their representatives, have shown the need to tax everyone more and more. This amounts to granting more governmental controls on everything, mostly us. Most Democratic governors have turned the way our major cities approve cost-cutting moves to defund police, replace justice with lawlessness, and replace political discussions with protesters burning cities down. Lest we forget, the beginnings of turning our former major cities' tourism trade into tent cities started in 2017 with their sanctuary-cities policy. Why did they do these things? It was for the sake of doing what the party leadership said to do. That is *take them cities down*. Me and my simple-minded approach from those observations were reminiscent of the old Red Armies of the Soviet Union in 1917 and of early Communist China in 1947. The radicals back then were also "activists." They believed in revolution at any price. God could not even help the death and destruction brought on by that ideology. Therefore, it is only fitting and logical to bring back the glory of the color red, as in the Red Army to radical left socialists and their "progressiveness" that now rules the "old Democratic Party." Please bring back the color red for the states that want to continue down that road of socialist "progressiveness."

Keeping with the color mapping of states, there are three states that do not fit into categories of either red, blue, or even purple states (swing states). They are the states of California, New York, and Illinois. Their colors should be blinking yellow caution lights. I base this observation on the fact that if governments are businesses, and they do try to maintain fiduciary responsibilities and budgeting. These states' runaway debt has earned them a blinking yellow light for caution. The citizens can begin to take control of their problems. First, stop voting in radical governors and other key representatives. You should begin to notice a significant turnaround in people's attitudes and financial bottom line. Why would this happen? It would happen because the people would start to believe in their leadership and the plan to move their states forward again instead of backward.

I believe our history books, if left untouched by WOKE ideology to change them, will show that President Donald Trump will go down in our history as one of the greatest presidents. That is whether he is able to seek another term in office in 2024 or not. His legacy will be that the American major media outlets and their political news outlets never let up on him, giving him only "bad press," and made him mostly unable to do his job. The real legacy for Donald Trump may be as the greatest political martyr. It should be written in our history books the details of what dirty politics mean. It happens when powerful media giants and large corporations work together to stifle the work needed by our elected executives. They attempted to make it dysfunctional. Clearly not to make it better, but maybe even to take America down.

## OUR DEFENSE

Our country has a history of being attacked by adversaries, both from outside its borders and from within. An example within is Benedict Arnold, a convicted traitor due to payoffs. We should have read about most of our adversaries from our history books. It started with the British from our nation's birth, with our Declaration of Independence and then the War of 1812. Later there was the Mexican War, the Civil War, the Spanish-American War, WWI, WWII, the Korean War, and the recent conflicts. They often say in sports that the best defense is a good offense. Being a sports enthusiast, I can relate to that. Every American must understand that a democracy is a very fragile form of government when compared to the authoritarian or command systems of totalitarianism (communism/socialism), nationalism, imperialism, and dictatorships. Therefore, because these authoritarian countries still exist, practicing democracies like ours must be continually on the alert.

Authoritarian governments need control over their people. They feel that real working, effective democracies like ours, with the participative role of their people, destroy their objective of total control, especially if it's a long-range goal for world domination. Therefore, the real democracies are targeted as adversaries. Citizen participation dilutes their authority and may spark demonstrations by their people for more freedoms in their countries. It happened in the failed USSR and presently is happening in Hong Kong. A major point for those command systems is to avoid any world news cameras showing either their people being disappointed in their leadership, or worse, demonstrating. For communist socialists, it is detrimental to their philosophy, because socialism is their promised nirvana.

There are examples of our own citizenry taking arms against our laws. I mentioned Benedict Arnold. We also had Shays' Rebellion over unpopular taxes in Massachusetts, and also John Brown's incitement at Harpers Ferry, Virginia, over slavery. Externally there was the attack by the British on our initial thirteen colonies.

The British in the late 1700s and into the 1800s were building an empire. The American colonies were a significant source for raw materials, clothing, and military supplies, furthering their empire's expansion. The Mexican American War was the result of an attack by Mexico, fundamentally over a territorial dispute. Our Civil War was caused by the powerful elitists in our southern states to maintain slavery, their utmost economic resource to maintain their economic status.

World War I was touched off by a European empire's suppression of its people and the assassination of the Austro-Hungarian Empire's Archduke Ferdinand. When Germany sank the *Lusitania*, killing American citizens, it justified our entry into that war.

World War II was started by dictators from Germany and the USSR, both invading a free, democratic but vulnerable Poland. The United States entered that war because of the Japanese Empire's attack at Pearl Harbor. Japan's reasoning for the attack was the same as the British Empire's war with us. The United States stopped trading critical raw materials to Japan. Those materials were needed to fuel their military expansion, specifically their war with Nationalist China.

Our latest conflicts have been caused by zealot-radical ideology. The conflicts in Korea and Vietnam were due to the socialist communists' manifesto for world domination. Radical religious beliefs led to the 9/11 attack and the destruction of the Twin Towers in New York City.

This chapter's section on defense is not intended to encourage you to turn the United States into a hi-tech weapons factory that could further torch our beautiful planet. Its purpose is to understand and value our democratic system of participative government, which places us as the greatest country in the world. However, it generates envy and even hatred from other countries. Everyone should take the time to notice the destruction of our major cities through increased crime and drug use. These are the results of political leaders that foster dividing the good people of our nation by creating hate instead of love and respect for each other. That ideology gets them votes from some bases, but cripples the bonds we share to preserve our nation.

It is not the amount of military weaponry needed for our defense. It is more the understanding that *our* adversaries are using our great democracy itself as the tool to defeat us. Why should our adversaries spend billions of dollars on military weaponry to defeat us? The Union of Soviet Socialist Republics (USSR) tried to do it by amassing military armaments until they went bankrupt. Their military plans failed, their people revolted, and the USSR failed and collapsed. *It is less costly for our adversaries to beat us by alienating our own people against each other.* Simply stated, that is what is really happening in America now. While the people of our nation are distracted by the current trends of online buying and streaming, our adversaries are taking advantage to defeat our democracy, which IS our nation's birthright. Our great democracy itself is being used as a weapon by controlling forces. It is a result of democracy's inherent DNA for its people to have the ability to spite the hand that feeds them. Looking back at our world's history, the French Revolution that took place in 1789 did take the French monarchy down. However, the social chaos during the aftermath of the revolution led to Napoleon Bonaparte becoming their dictator. Today, authoritarians do not need a one-person dictator. Their group of highly organized "smarties" can agree to do the same thing, only with more combined technical resources. What are we going to do to  keep our country's birthright safe?  We have to work harder and smarter and pay attention to our country's business of keeping our borders safe and our budget controllable.

Historically, it was our great manufacturing ability that led us to victories in both world wars. Without a manufacturing base we would have been unable to produce the necessary tools and equipment for our defense. Do we use our plastic credit cards with their ever-increasing cycle of national debt to purchase defense items from Communist China like we do with everything else? The country that monetarily benefited the most from the COVID-19 pandemic was, coincidentally, where the virus came from. China was there to help our pandemic-filled world with billions of masks and disinfectants FOR SALE! What a big-hearted nation. Herein lies our problem. I hope you can see how defenseless we are. We must fix this security problem! We must return to manufacturing our own products that have real value. Well-made equipment is essential for our defense. This equipment must not fail as often as the poorly made online products we have recently been purchasing from overseas. I suppose you were unaware of that fact. Read the labels. Practically everything in our stores, including online stores, is made in China.

I cannot emphasize enough how many in Congress want to take every nickel that they can from your wallets and purses. It is not for our nation's defense to be sure. Believe me, many would rather cut that budget, like the Clinton administration did, and have more money for the politicians to play with. That action weakened our defense back then and it led to the 9/11 disaster. They want the power (money) to dole it out, not necessarily for their constituents, but to lobbyists and their campaign contributors. They want the money in their hands and not *your* hands. They only want to keep the middle class "sustainable"—actually monetarily "controllable"—at best. Heaven forbid, should you have more of your income available, you may even do the unthinkable and enroll your children in private schools rather than public schools.

About twenty years ago the people I worked with in a business building (not in our homes like today) would discuss the stock market and other important newsworthy topics of the day. It was a time when the stock market was on a real roller-coaster ride. I told them I used the stock market as a gauge as to how I was doing financially. I told them that when the stock market was doing good, I must be doing bad. Conversely, when the stock market is doing bad, I must be doing good. They asked how I arrived at that conclusion. I told them that I am a typical middle-class citizen. When the stock market is good that means they, the banks and investors, have my money. When the stock market is bad, that means I must be saving my money. I believe in our nation's investors. They will assure that the stock market will have continual growth. It is in their best interest to do so. However, I also care about the amount of money I save, for my family's sake. I care about how my savings institutions invest in the market. They are the experts, and I have always depended on their good judgment. I care about only spending enough for me or my family's needs, keeping vanity down, but giving rewards out when deserved. Relative to our defense, our government should be sponsoring bonds for our defense. At one time we called them war bonds. I believe we should be calling them defense bonds. Bonds are typically a financially safe way to save money and, in the case of our national defense, keep the industries that promote a great defense active. No matter who the president of the United States is, those bonds will assure a stream of resources to keep us safe.

This book's title is *2020 Visions: For Families, Friends, the Hopeful and the Helpful.* Your understanding of our adversaries, the hell-bent ideologies of special interest groups, and the wealth and power of others, is our best defense to save our democratic system of government. It is a fragile system. I am repeating myself, not to use condition response to trick you, but to drive home the importance of the Achilles' heel that democracy has. Please open your eyes, physically assemble with others, and discuss what is really happening here. It is your constitutional right to assemble, pandemic or not. Put honest representatives in office to regulate the hi-tech tools and mechanisms that are negatively affecting our naïve, unsuspecting people's minds. The understanding and knowledge of democracy itself, being used as a tool against itself, is our best defense against our free nation's adversaries. Discuss the issues that are affecting our nation. We are the great middle class and can fix our problems just as we always have. Take the time to be objective with all information that is presented to you as news. I said earlier in this book to take the time to gather information about a subject before deciding on it. A paramount change that must happen for our defense is the reestablishing of manufacturing in this country. It not only positions us to manufacture defensive tools, but also promotes higher-paying wages for our people. It will help families to help pay off costly college loans for instance. Let's face the realities that a college education has not fulfilled the promise of creating significant increases in wages for the middle class.

## CHAPTER RESTROSPECTIVE

When I started writing this book in 2017 and '18, I started picking out topics from my recent observations. They totaled thirty different topics. That meant thirty chapters. The book's editor advised me to trim that down. He said that was too much for one reader to take on. I agreed, but then I had to decide which chapters to merge. The easiest four chapters to merge became this chapter. Our government, with the way it operates or does not operate today, became the perfect one to merge. This chapter easily combined economics, politics, and our defense with government. They are all neatly tied together in one nice package. I always say everything is a business, and how we run as a business will make us or break us. It is especially important for us, the great middle class, to know and understand how we spend our tax money.

During my career in government my colleagues and I would always fall back on the term *proven effective methods*. You must remember that there are 535 people in Congress trying to run our government, or at the very least legislate (our laws). The people in Congress come from a variety of backgrounds, cultures, education, and experiences. They know they are placed in a circumstance for diplomacy and try to reach

a common ground on issues. Consensus is the objective in their important committees. Hence, this is the problem. If you have leadership that
has little knowledge on complex matters and reaches a consensus, they
may be technically wrong when trying to put it into practice. They have
the power and authority to start a venture, but never take the time to
pre-test it before initiating it. This occurs because they hurriedly inform
their constituents about the issue's progress. Project dates for fixing
issues are established without regard for the number of details, like testing, which need to take place for important projects. Believe me, those
details can be real showstoppers. Again, the rule of thumb is to use
proven effective methods and to evaluate certain methods to see how
they would fit and function for an issue. Then grade these results. If our
country's leadership started doing more of this, we would be in a safer
and better economic state. Issues like high inflation, recessions, or security issues could be avoided.

Our legislators are voted in to legislate! We constantly hear that there
is too much regulation. For the well-being of our nation, legislators must
legislate! That is what they are elected to do. It wasn't to tape TV interviews for their personal feelings on personal matters or party platforms.
Our legislators can see how party platforms easily divide our nation. It's
just not a constructive idea to continually fan the flames of those differences instead of working on issues that benefit our nation. This chapter on
government, economics, politics, and defense is one reason why I wrote
this book. Our legislators, paid with our tax money (hopefully only with
our tax money, and not lobbyists or political ideologists), are there to lead.
They should allow for a growing economy, to police corruption, and to
keep our nation safe with a strong defense. If Congress does that it will
lead to smiles on the faces of their customers, their constituents. Our
nation was built on and for democracy. Killing our democracy will kill our
nation. I often said in this book that we must choose our leadership more
carefully. Someone may look the part of a politician but that's not any

reason to elect them. I wonder how much better our government would be if we elected more librarians.

I have observed that I really don't think most people are in control of anything anymore, let alone their income. The sad thing is that many of the things that run our nation are at the top on the political triangle or pyramid seen in figure 17-B. The best way for the citizenry to control our nation is to get our legislators, the electorate we chose, to regulate them. Teddy Roosevelt, a progressive in his day, did that over a hundred years ago, and now we must do it again. It is time for the real "democracy" Democrats and Republicans to assemble, as when our nation was formed under Thomas Jefferson, and put the power of our democracy back into the hands of the middle class. When I worked in government, I had a sign posted in my office that said, *If you are not part of the solution, YOU are part of the problem.*

Due to the number of topics, the music that inspired me to write this chapter came from five songs. They are "Ball of Confusion," performed by the Temptations and written by Norman Whitfield and Barrett Strong; "The Pusher," performed by Steppenwolf and written by Hoyt Wayne Axton; "Backstabbers," performed by the O'Jays and written by Leon Huff, Gene McFadden, and John Whitehead; "Taxman," performed by the Beatles and written by George Harrison; and "Sixteen Tons," performed by Tennessee Ernie Ford and written by Merle Travis.

The Temptations are singing about social issues that occurred in the 1960s and still exist today. They are things like cities being set on fire like in 2020, the sale of dangerous drugs, gun control, our education system, and my favorite, where politicians insist that more taxes will solve everything. How have supposedly educated Americans not resolved these issues in over fifty years? It may be that they could not reach a consensus about them, or that the issues themselves help keep alive the prospect that they can be used for election purposes. Our politicians should be graded on the issues they resolved, not on how good they made their constituents feel.

John Kaye of the rock group Steppenwolf sings about drug pushers. Today it is much more than that. Those little miniature Chinese billboard smartphones are keeping us away from the ability to digest issues and make good decisions. Every time a bell or buzz comes out of that thing, you are expected to react. Instead of being the person to manage each issue and then prioritize it, you end up being like a telephone switchboard operator. Unfortunately for you, unlike that old telephone switchboard operator, you do not have a cord to grab and delay any action on them. The device expects you to react to the alert. DO YOU REALLY HAVE THE TIME FOR ALL THAT CLUTTER? You do not, and no one does. Years ago, when managers had secretaries answering their phone, they would instruct them to tell the sales caller, "We do not want any." For other calls they would answer, "Do not call us, we will call you!" That took care of the clutter back then.

In "Backstabbers," the O'Jays sing about people, and I paraphrase, to watch out for smiling faces. They say that all the time. They also say others just want to take your place, and if you really care you had better beware. They are singing about the shady characters in the world when they say their fists are tight and their blades are long and aimed straight at your back. The song reminds me of how Henry Kessinger went to Communist China in 1971 to build a relationship, and we saw smiling faces from an impoverished nation and began trade relations with them. As a sign of friendship and goodwill back then, they even gave us panda bears. Now in the twenty-first century all they want to do is to dominate the world by sticking a knife in our back, and at a time when we were economically down due to a worldwide pandemic that came from, none the less, China.

In the song "Taxman," George Harrison wrote about how the government, and I paraphrase, will tell YOU how it will be. They'll tax you and give you back about 5 percent of the 100 percent you expect from them. If you drive a car, they'll tax the street; if you are cold, they'll tax the heat. If you walk, they will even tax your feet. It sounds like a great book or movie that Dr. Seuss could have created. George ends with his point that the pennies you earned in life should be carefully invested, because if you don't you will be giving your earnings to a governmental body that wants it all.

In the song "Sixteen Tons," Tennessee Ernie Ford sings and I paraphrase again, another day older and deeper in debt. That is because he is working in a coal mine and the coal company coincidentally owns the only store in town, they can and do control all of the store's products. They have the pricing inflated enough so the singer can never get ahead, because they also control his meager wages. It comes to a point where he is not getting ahead and even working longer hours. He explains that for him, the reason he is getting further in debt is because his work, which he calls his soul, is owned by the company store. I see how this can be related to our government and economics so as to kill our middle class, the hardworking middle class that is trying very hard to get out of debt.

"Sixteen Tons" could also be construed as an example of the dichotomy of the past two centuries. However, it is meant to have people understand two important points, regardless of the two centuries. The first point is to fully comprehend the many hardships most Americans worked and suffered through to build this giant beacon for liberty, freedom, and democracy called "America."

The second point is about greed and controlling, powerful people in large industries and in government. They cannot help their greedy, selfish affliction. These hucksters have created an unholy alliance of the biggest corporations, their advertising media, and elected officials and want to control the world's money supply. They do this by spinning their sticky tentacles on the internet, coincidentally called the worldwide web, which is technically a monopoly. It is a monopoly because commerce is conducted on it and there is only one internet.

"Sixteen Tons" is a song about coal miners and the tyranny the mine owners held over their employees and the entire mining community. The mine owners controlled the town. They controlled the banks, bars, hotels, housing, stores, and even the local sheriff and deputies. The miners, their families, and everyone in the town was subjected to control by the mine owners. The worst part was that the company store was owned by the mine company. It was a requirement by the mine owners that all the equipment and uniforms needed by miners be purchased from the company store. There were no options to purchase goods anywhere else, because competition was not allowed. There were no other stores for miles around to purchase any goods, even food and clothing. These items were conveniently shelved at the company store. For the miners it seemed that the harder and longer they worked for more income, the more the prices at the company store, and the rent they paid for the homes owned by the mine owners, kept going up. The mine owners kept making more of a profit on the town's people. People should not—no, can never—allow themselves to be in a position to be economically controlled by one source, or worse, by a cartel of swindlers. Freedom-loving people always need a ready source of options, or competition, to the "company stores" of our world.

These songs make me understand why our younger population has become so angry. Surely they should see that internet buying from one main source, and the internet itself, is a monopoly, and only gives those companies using it more power to control marketplaces. This act limits competition and does not offer any solutions to raising wages for those working in those organizations unless they are unionized. It isn't any wonder why this generation has so little faith in our nation's future.

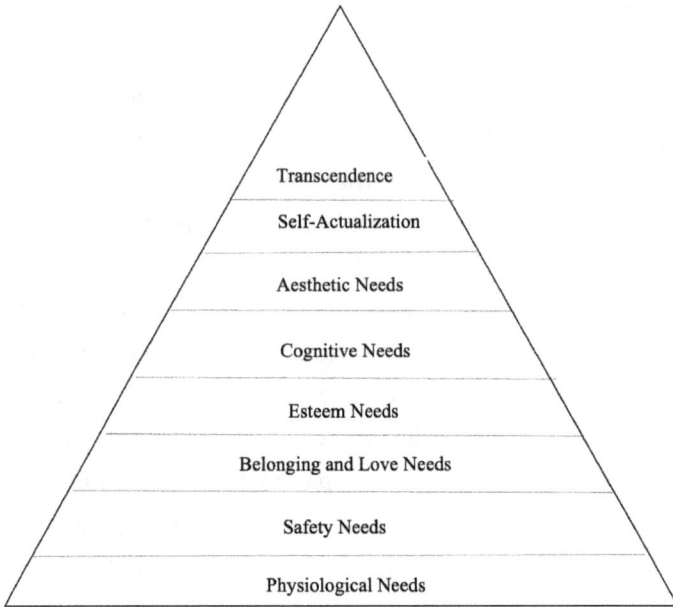

**Maslow's Hierarchy of Needs**

Fig. 17-A

# THE POLITICAL TRIANGLE OR PYRAMID IN AMERICA

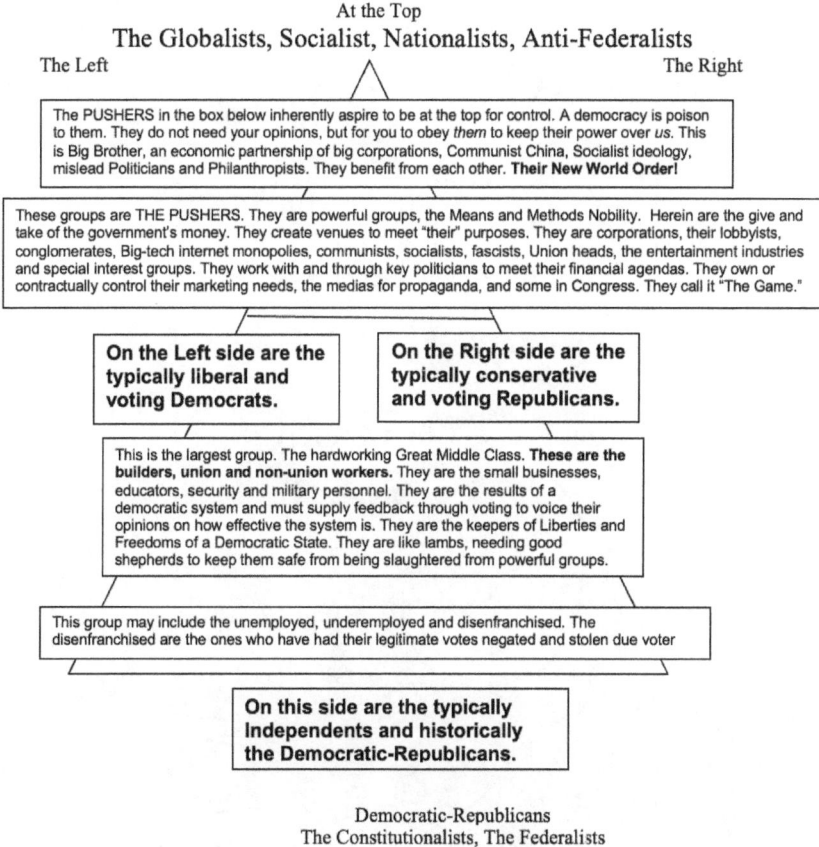

At the Top
## The Globalists, Socialist, Nationalists, Anti-Federalists

The Left ⟋⟍ The Right

The PUSHERS in the box below inherently aspire to be at the top for control. A democracy is poison to them. They do not need your opinions, but for you to obey *them* to keep their power over *us*. This is Big Brother, an economic partnership of big corporations, Communist China, Socialist ideology, mislead Politicians and Philanthropists. They benefit from each other. **Their New World Order!**

These groups are THE PUSHERS. They are powerful groups, the Means and Methods Nobility. Herein are the give and take of the government's money. They create venues to meet "their" purposes. They are corporations, their lobbyists, conglomerates, Big-tech internet monopolies, communists, socialists, fascists, Union heads, the entertainment industries and special interest groups. They work with and through key politicians to meet their financial agendas. They own or contractually control their marketing needs, the medias for propaganda, and some in Congress. They call it "The Game."

| **On the Left side are the typically liberal and voting Democrats.** | **On the Right side are the typically conservative and voting Republicans.** |

This is the largest group. The hardworking Great Middle Class. **These are the builders, union and non-union workers.** They are the small businesses, educators, security and military personnel. They are the results of a democratic system and must supply feedback through voting to voice their opinions on how effective the system is. They are the keepers of Liberties and Freedoms of a Democratic State. They are like lambs, needing good shepherds to keep them safe from being slaughtered from powerful groups.

This group may include the unemployed, underemployed and disenfranchised. The disenfranchised are the ones who have had their legitimate votes negated and stolen due voter

**On this side are the typically Independents and historically the Democratic-Republicans.**

Democratic-Republicans
The Constitutionalists, The Federalists

Fig. 17–B

165

## The Tornado Triangle or Swirly Created at a Democracy's Demise

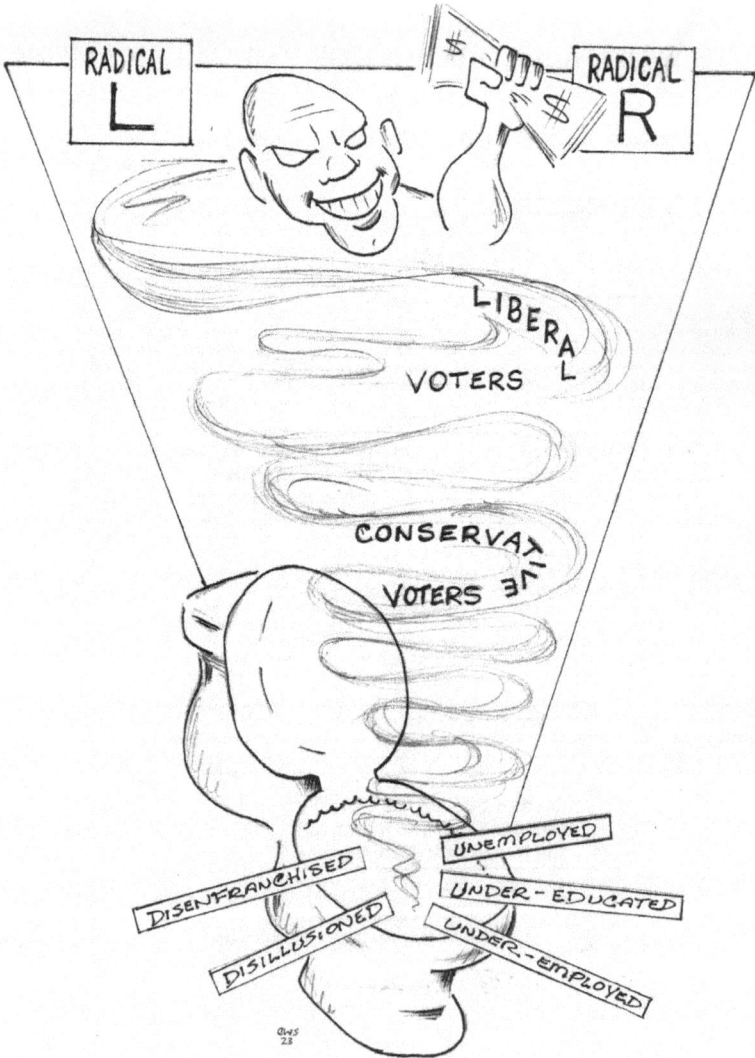

Figure 17-C

The Swirly happens when business partnerships with the Communist-Socialists and the world's largest corporations take hold. Their objective is to control the markets and money, killing the middle class and their ability to financially do anything about it. The result is that citizens feel handcuffed and treated as slaves. The lowest on Maslow's Hierarchy of Needs are the first to go down the tubes. The wealthiest, with unpatriotic business dealings, believe they will be freed from the tube.

# 18.

# Our Health, Diet, Environment and Pollution

This chapter covers the topics of our health, diet, environment, and pollution. I'm writing this in the early spring of 2022. That is two and a half years from the onset of the COVID-19 virus as it was reported from Communist China. At this writing, our world is still feeling the effects of the pandemic. The experts cautioned in early 2020 that it may last up to four years. I envisioned this pandemic to be as destructive to the world's economy as the 1930s depression was. If not the world's economy, at least the United States economy. I believe I was not alone in that belief, and therefore Congress appropriated monetary relief for certain groups. After this lab incident there has not been an economic depression, but maybe worse, irretrievable damage to our minds, bodies, and the overall health of our nation. The pandemic has affected our daily norms. We acquire norms to help us make purposeful decisions, and as a defense mechanism. People generally adapt to changes, but inherently become resistant to changes when their many norms are compromised. Established norms permit periods of security, self-confidence, and tranquility. They allow for rational behavior as issues arise.

## OUR MENTAL AND BEHAVIORAL HEALTH

[1]Let us look at how norms are defined by a dictionary. A norm is:
1. An authoritative standard: MODEL.
2. A principle of right action binding upon members of a

group and serving to guide, control, or regulate proper and acceptable behavior.

3. AVERAGE: A) as a set standard of development or achievement usually. B) a pattern or trait taken to be typical in the behavior of a social group.

Have you thought about how we all were herded into our homes and away from our previously direct face-to-face assemblies due to the COVID-19 pandemic? I hope you have given that some thought. It may be history for you, but we should have learned a lesson from that experience. Many of our established American norms have been *turned upside down* by COVID. Before COVID, people wearing masks were considered bandits or thieves. Although at one time netted veils over women's hats were customary, especially during periods of mourning. The pandemic caused many mask-wearing people to be heroic (and rightly so) in the healthcare industry. Other groups used mask wearing as an opportunity to burn buildings and cause anarchy. They seized mask wearing as a spineless tool so as not to be recognized in public. COVID caused the discontinuance of any public signs of friendship such as shaking hands or hugs. There was a standing order to stay back six feet from human faces that were most probably not smiling. Our homes, *our safe houses*, were turned into school classrooms and workspaces. The pandemic negated most religious rituals, workplace discussions, and maybe most importantly, altered your former shopping routines. The destruction of private or government property previously was considered a crime. Opportunists were calling that destruction and terror a justice-based necessity. They gave no thought to the fact that somebody, probably the middle-class insurance holders, had to pay for the damage with higher premium costs. Some disconnected state governors called the summer of 2020 the "summer of love." The most serious effect was that the police became bad people, *the ones who were formerly cast as the officer friendlies in our elementary schools*. I suppose opportunists welcomed the thought of turning crime prevention into "Dodge City" justice and establishing a new set of norms. In essence, the maskless face-to-face discussions with real people in public became almost nil. There was practically no discussion about anyone's thoughts about "what's goin' on" during the COVID-19 onslaught. Any discussions were considered unnecessary, baseless lecturing creating dangerous puffs of diseased vapor with every word. Yes, I did use the word *opportunists* when describing some people's actions and their "appreciation" for the pandemic. The word *opportunists* here is meant in the most despicable sense. Some people may have even thought it was an opportunity to rid our country of its standing president.

The COVID-19 pandemic caused changes to our norms. Herding us into our homes required us to use virtual ideology (not technology) in our supposedly personal and private dwellings. *Virtual is not reality.* [2]A dictionary defines *virtual* as 1) being such in essence or effect though not formally recognized or admitted; or 2) of, relating to, or using virtual memory.

Prolonged participation in virtual activities can cause a disconnect with people because the images are not real (non-three-dimensional), and LCD screens *limit viewing* to making viewers only focus on the presenter's setting instead of an entire scene or classroom, for example. Our school children who had to suffer though this norm change and its muffled communication probably now feel more secure using electronic tools than face-to-face communications. This may be because those tools provide clearer interpretation of lessons rather than muffled tones from their teachers. So, if your children seem to be put off by real face-to-face discussions these days, it is because their communication "norm" has changed. It seems that our children are always the forgotten ones though the hard times. For some powerful groups, the pandemic and those mentioned changes to our norms must have been like manna from heaven. The groups I am alluding to are the ones that did large amounts of technical-device sales to families and schools that had to purchase more of these devices. The real big bene-factor of the hi-tech-tools sales ended up being the foreign nations that manufactured them and the few large suppliers of them.

During these norm changes you may have been naively ignoring your health because of the new public mandates thrust upon you. Your physical and mental health has been affected and is *still being tested*. Presently many are struggling to deal with the stress of increased inflation and higher costs for energy, utilities, food and everything else. Our once-great American middle class is feeling these stressful challenges and trying to cope with all of them.

Through COVID, the many sheltered-in-place Americans were receiving compensation for being unemployed. They were left watching TV screens and smartphones for the latest COVID updates and, coinci-dentally, the politics of the 2020 election. From my observations the pan-demic created an outburst of a mentally degenerative disease called com-pulsive buying disorder (CBD). Our TV, computers, and smartphones are littered with a constant stream of advertising. Let's face it, there is far too much advertising of everything today. They are on all roadside billboards, all sporting arenas, hair salons, and even our clothing. Even the Major League Baseball umpires' uniforms have an advertising logo on them. The company chosen for those uniforms is in an investment industry which has an unproven and scary track record.

Unfortunately, due to CDC recommendations, the pandemic forced an increase in internet usage on smartphones and computers which *made people* "electronically connected" more than ever. The stay-at-home man-dates directly caused an increased spike in CBD. The trend in internet use has tripled since 2009. *Yes, tripled.* In 2009 through 2011, much of internet usage was for research and the growth of social media. Online buying has soared an additional 50.5 percent since 2019, from the start of COVID-19 to the present. The pandemic *has directly created* a buying frenzy and problems for people oblivious to CBD.

In early 2022, the president's administration said that America was having a "supply chain problem." Every TV viewer in America saw the many giant freight containers lying idle on the West Coast shoreline. In reality, America was not having a supply chain problem, we were and are still having a *demand* chain problem. It is called CBD. The data suggests the pandemic from China caused this increase. The sad part about all this is that people in this country *and the world* will not, and probably cannot, stop themselves from online CBD. Unfortunately, due to the fact that it is a disorder, it affects our country's health. Government regulations are needed to monitor CBD, because it is affecting the growth of real equity.

Most everyone considered the required standing-order mandates to control the pandemic's spread a temporary disruption to their previous, normal way of life. Unfortunately, after three years, the "pandemic effect' has changed us. It may affect how others, even our government, may tolerate your acceptance of the new norms. There are articles about social norms and what is called *deviance*—going against new norms—on the internet. It is a little frightening because clearly the pandemic has affected our previous comfortable norms and transitioned many into uncomfortable new norms. The deviance to those new norms by you is directly attributed to the pandemic's required social mandates. Many just press on with these new altered routines, accepting them because we keep telling ourselves they are only temporary.

Many of the pandemic effects have created other norms. For instance, when the COVID levels are near zero, even in warmer weather, many people continually wear masks. I can only surmise that it is some form of identity group telegraphing that they are *all in* with all the new social changes from COVID that many keep touting. The science says that wearing masks for an extended period of time causes mask-induced exhaustion syndrome (MIES). MIES has been identified as gene-altering and linked to embryonic development and cancer. Additionally, there are ongoing studies on how depleted amounts of oxygen from mask wearing can affect the brain and other organs. As a test, hold your breath for a period of time and tell me how you feel.

I will try to help those that may have anxieties over these pandemic social changes (the point of new norms versus old norms). Former President Ronald Reagan may have given us the answer. He addressed the American TV audience many times with this quote: "Right has might." If you feel that previous norms were more emotionally calming and comforting than the recent changes confronting you, go with what you know is the right thing to do. Hopefully, spiritually and maybe scientifically those old norms are *proven effective methods*. Right does have might.

From my observations I see smartphones, TV, the internet, and their advertisers as nothing more than herding devices no different than cattle prodders or tasers. The only difference is that, instead of stinging you, they are like an addictive drug. They affect our brain endorphins, as well as our ability to pay for the damage and expense they cause. When doing things that attract you to them but are harmful, it is like the old salesmanship teaching, "You can catch more flies with honey than you do with vinegar." Therefore, people get lured when they see products advertised by smiling actors and the gimmicks that go along with them. It is easy to get hooked, and you may also provide your credit card account numbers to hackers.

I have a tip for people with anxieties over the pandemic effects. Reduce your smartphone, gaming, and computer use. If you are continually walking around with a smartphone in your hand, you are missing out on a lot of what's going on around you in our natural world. Specifically, the 360-degree panoramic view of it. It is not that these devices are unhealthy, but *everything* should be done in moderation. These devices are a *distraction* from the wonderful real world we live in. You may have an addiction problem with these devices, much like kleptomania, gambling, or an eating disorder. To add insult to injury, almost all TV commercials since the pandemic show an actor with a smartphone in their hand to entice us to pick up "our tool," that we basically rent, and immediately order their advertised item.

Have you given any thought to the increase in personal storage containers over the past twenty-five years? Why is this? I do not own one and wonder what could possibly cause someone to rent one. I know people move and many times need someplace to store things between moves. However, there is an increase in storage containers used just to keep things. I hope that Americans are not becoming "closet" hoarders. People with CBD cannot help themselves. There are TV shows that show how some people are outwardly hoarding, but the increase in storage containers may be masking a real problem that our nation is facing today.

Many smartphones come with programs built in to show their amount of use. Whatever the amount is, set a figure of 50 percent of your current use and make it your new goal to limit its use to this amount of time. Do not look at the decreased use as merely a goal but a discovery of new activities with your newfound time. Record these new discoveries in a text or email to yourself. Write down any new and enjoyable people you have met or places you visited and things you did. It can be your diary or log. Add smiling emojis as needed. Help to build a world full of smiles, laughter, music, and dancing. It has been our heritage to be a fun-loving nation. Let's keep that tradition. These activities can help relieve us from life's mental frustrations. Play your favorite music through those handheld hypnotic devices, or better yet a radio, instead of purchasing things you probably do not need. While listening to that music, add a little dancing to it. Dancing is great exercise.

## OUR PHYSICAL HEALTH

There is an old adage that goes, "If you have your health, you have everything." Pain or other abnormalities effect your ability to function as you would like to. Are you an American? Your health not only affects you but our whole nation. We need you, even though you may *feel unwanted* because you do not fit any popular group's profile today. However, you are a big part of our nation's team plan. In team building it is important for each member to be as good as they can be. When every team member begins to work together it creates a well-oiled team of dynamos.

I do not know how the pandemic affected your preventive health needs. It affected my annual physical checkups. There was no way I or my wife were going into hospitals or health clinics with the potentially deadly COVID-19 spreading. That was a decision I am sure many others made as well. When we received our COVID vaccines it was a relief to be able to continue most of the pre-COVID activities that we had. My wife is an avid swimmer, and it was nice to see her renewed her passion for it. As for me, at over seventy, I was just happy to continue with my annual physicals and see my doctors to deal will the usual bumps and bruises that come with getting older.

Our country has been trying to control rising healthcare costs since they began to balloon in the 1990s. However, it never happened. Perhaps the healthcare industry did not want those rising healthcare costs to consumers being fixed. There is nothing like the status quo to maintain revenues. However, the healthcare customers, which most Americans are, want to *lower healthcare costs!* Families or individuals need options as to where their money is invested or spent. People have to pay for home mortgages or rent, quality (choice) education for themselves and their children, retirement investments, and utility expenses.

Past federal administrations were successful in insuring Americans got their meds. The pharmaceutical industry began to take off like a rocket in the 1990s. Most of the medications people take today are needed because their bodies are breaking down from not getting enough exercise, eating/drinking properly, or getting at least six to seven hours of continuous sleep (hopefully during the night). It is best to keep a steady balance of healthy food and safe drinking water, moderate exercise, and a consistent amount of sleep *every day*. I have a fact for you: Most drugs are harmful to your body. The human organs like kidneys, livers, and pancreases cannot handle large amounts or mixtures of drugs. If you do not feel those effects immediately, you will see their effects later in life.

My mother was a prime example of how drugs can cause irreparable damage. She started to see a doctor about her depression in her late sixties. My father died at age fifty-five and left her heartbroken and lonely. So, her loss caused her depression, and her doctor prescribed meds for her. At her next physical checkup, she learned she had a touch of diabetes. So, diabetes meds were prescribed. At her next medical evaluation, they discovered she had high blood pressure; therefore, meds were prescribed. Sometime later they discovered she had high cholesterol. Once again, meds were prescribed for this as well. As a family we tried in vain to keep all those different meds straight. At some time in her seventies, my mother passed out on the kitchen floor from being over-medicated. At that point, short-term memory loss and dementia began. My mother was never the same after that. She ended up in a nursing home until the age of ninety-three. Too much medication, or worse, combinations of medications, may damage your body's immune system. Once that system begins to break down it cannot fight off viruses, bacteria, or even food allergies to begin repairing itself.

I suppose I'll never understand the logic for the individual health tax mandated in the Affordable Care Act. That tax was a whopping $350 to $500 per-month expense for most Americans. I found it ridiculous for single people without families, between the ages of twenty-six and forty-five, in the prime of their life, to be *told they must have healthcare*. To me it was like the Mafia telling people they had to pay for "their protection." People don't need healthcare until they *need* healthcare. Between the ages of twenty-six and forty-five is typically the time for families to begin their planning for growth. It is a time for home buying, building equity for families, and investing in retirement funds. To take that exceedingly high amount of money away from that bracket of Americans every month for healthcare and pharmaceuticals is an economic drain. It alters the savings for home buying and other forms of proven, smart equity building, as well as everyone's financial security, which definitely affects the economic health of a nation.

## A HEALTHY DIET

Cleary we are what we eat. Like our computer instructors tell us: Garbage in, garbage out! Keep a regimen of a good diet, which contains a balance of the five food groups. Follow those rules and eat that balance of foods in moderation. Eating too little doesn't feed our mind and body cells the nutrients they need. Eating too much causes obesity. Our foods, exercise, and social activities affect us. All of those activities listed make for a better YOU. The five food groups are:

1. Fruits and vegetables
2. Carbohydrates from grains or starch (potatoes and pasta)
3. Proteins from meats and poultry, fish, eggs, tofu, and nuts
4. Dairy from milk, yogurt, cheese, or alternatives—mostly reduced fat
5. Fats and sugars from oils and sweets

Fresh fruits or vegetables are preferred over canned foods. Feeding our body's cells with fresh nutrients keeps our digestive system naturally regular. In order to prevent certain types of cancer, it's important to eat foods that contain fiber. The saying "garbage in, garbage out" applies here. Keeping our body's garbage can (the colon) clean is important too. If you don't like eating whole wheat breads and cereals, substitute them with foods containing beans, like chili. Limit your intake of red meat to one or two times per week. Eating fresh fish at least once a week rounds out your diet for proteins. Stay away from protein product supplements. They are not fresh proteins and contain milk byproducts. When eating grains, try eating oat cereals, hot or cold, at least two times a week. Oats are not only good for your heart but provide muscle strength. Keep your lungs free from smoke or anything that pollutes the air. We have already discussed the overuse of masking.

If you are experiencing abnormal symptoms like diarrhea, blisters, or constant headaches, see your doctor. You may have an allergy to certain foods. In 2007, my wife was hospitalized for three days due to the symptoms of a stroke. After an analysis, her doctor determined that she may have had a reaction to the MSG (monosodium glutamate) from a restaurant's soup she had eaten earlier that day. Later we found out she does have an MSG issue.

MSG is a dangerous food additive. One week after my wife's hospital stay, she had similar symptoms. She had eaten a particular brand of cheese puff curls and had a reaction. Her face started to feel like ants were crawling all over it, and she began to get dizzy. My son read the ingredients list and verified the cheese curls had the ingredient MSG. Since these episodes, my wife and I always read labels, not just on food but on everything.

After that unfortunate MSG issue, my wife started to experience stomach pains and blisters on her hands. After visits to determine the cause, doctors recommended that she have her gall bladder removed, have a milk allergy, irritable bowel syndrome (IBS), and may have anxiety issues. They also said that the blisters may be eczema. After all their guess work I would definitely have an anxiety issue. At about that same time I was searching for a New-York-style pizza dough on the internet. I kept seeing popup advertisements for GLUTEN-FREE. I did not know anything about it. I read articles about people with allergies to wheat gluten and celiac disease. One article showed a photo of a woman's blistered hands from the effects of eating wheat gluten. They looked just like my wife's blistered hands. I showed the photo to my wife. She immediately stopped eating foods containing wheat, barley, and rye. For years after that, her hand blisters and stomach pains went away. Over twenty years of constant bouts of diarrhea went away as well.

As you may be aware, some chemicals give off dangerous odors. One most people should be concerned with is cookware with non-stick coatings. Research has proven that cooking with some of these products causes pet-bird deaths. Also, there are as many as six toxic gasses released by them. We use stainless and porcelain-coated cookware in our home. They clean fairly easily when lightly greased or buttered and heated over moderate heat before placing food in them.

Many years ago, my family went on a Florida vacation. One park had a pavilion dedicated to modern farming techniques. The attraction was all about our land. It included human interaction with our earth. Also, inside the exhibit was an attraction about the foods we eat. It featured a talking refrigerator with rap music in the background. The refrigerator told the importance of reading food wrappers and understanding their nutritional value. Its intent was for people to read food labels and to be concerned about the ingredients and additives in them. People should be cognizant of what they are eating. You would be surprised by how many unhealthy or unnecessary chemicals are in processed food. Eat healthier, eat more fresh foods and less "fast foods" and processed or prepared foods. READ THE LABELS.

I learned some important farming techniques from a 1947 movie titled *Give Us the Earth*. It is a wonderful documentary about the work of Dr. Spencer Hatch. He and his wife worked with a very poor, small Mexican village to correct their farming deficiencies. The village's subsistence was based on farming. These villagers did not use any modern farming techniques. Their soil was burnt out from a lack of crop rotation and other issues. Even their livestock suffered through their poor farming methods. It took all the energy of Dr. Hatch and his wife to get the villagers to clear their prejudices about Americans and "buy into" newer farming techniques. Eventually the villagers began to understand how he and his wife were there in earnest. These farming villagers had only themselves and hope and prayers for their crops and lives to improve. Through Dr. Hatch's work he turned mostly wasted land into a breadbasket and a horn of plenty. The foods produced were all natural from naturally produced amendments. As the livestock began to eat better, they produced many other necessary food groups, like milk and meat, for a better balanced diet within the community. Eating fresh foods that your own hands produce from the earth is so rewarding. Consider growing a garden or going fishing for some fresh food. Being close to nature, our land and streams, makes people feel like protecting them. It is not surprising that when people get out of the big cities and visit state and national parks they say, "I was out in God's Country."

## OUR ENVIRONMENT AND POLLUTION

I started to be an environmentalist, so to speak, at a very young age. Alex, a third-grade friend of mine, became a junior ranger for Smokey the Bear, therefore I became one too. I received materials about preventing forest fires and low-impact camping. The coolest part was the gold Smokey-the-Bear ranger badge I proudly wore. I don't know for sure how that affected my attitudes on our environment, but I never went out of my way to trash our environment, and neither did my father. When I was eleven years old, I took a hatchet from my dad's tool shed. I put a few cuts into a three-inch-diameter sassafras sapling. My dad took the hatchet from me and told me, "Never cut another tree down in the yard." He then took some wide tape and wrapped it around the damage I had made to the tree's bark.

In 1970, my senior year in high school, I joined an after-school program called Ecology Now. We worked on projects to rectify environmental issues. After all, Cleveland was known to be the first large metropolitan city in America to have a major river catch on fire. It was the Cuyahoga

River that runs through northeastern Ohio and feeds into Lake Erie. It caught fire due to all the chemical pollutants in it. That incident became a national joke for some time. The jokes bothered me because I had an appreciation for our environment.

I often wonder if Americans think about the increases in our rubbish collection over the last ten years. I mentioned our increased purchasing of overseas products and CBD. Do we ever give any thought to where these products end up after their use, or failure? They go into our rubbish, then to waste-material sites. I understand how these waste sites are manufactured with clay insulating materials; however, the combination of these materials seeping into our underground water tables is dangerous. We never think about our water tables because we don't see them.

I was blessed to have had a job driving the elderly and disabled to their medical appointments. That driving position allowed me to see the many streets and roads in and around the county where I live. I was amazed at how many residents have lawncare services for fertilizing and preventing weeds. I don't have this service, and in my over forty-five years of home ownership, I never have. I did and still do fertilize, but I stay away from unnatural pesticides. The chemicals that we put on our lawns eventually get into the water tables. They get washed into the sewer systems that feed our lakes. As an alternative for weed prevention, consider Zoysia japonica grass. It is sold by many seed-supply companies. This grass is so thick that it prevents weeds from poking through and is used by many golf courses.

Another concern I have relative to our water supply is the continued use of drugs by Americans. I am aware that many cities have programs where they will collect unused drugs. These drugs are then incinerated. However, my concern is that the ingested drugs (chemicals) are naturally being released by our bodies and end up being "flushed" so to speak. They absolutely end up in our sanitary sewer systems. The research shows that many of these chemicals *do not break down* in the water treatment plants. Therefore, they remain in our water supply system.

We often wonder why we have so many cases of cancer, birth defects, or autism. We see people with hormone, estrogen, and testosterone issues today. Could the increase in pharmaceuticals being taken since the mid-1990s have affected our genes through our water system? If we are what we eat or drink, our bodies could be reacting to all the chemicals in our freshwater systems. We have succeeded in lowering mercury levels in our water. However, it is time to remove all other chemicals as well!

After discussing how much I respect our environment, I believe the Green New Deal that the progressive socialists are pushing is a bad deal for America right now. First, our country and our world is still trying to pay off the debt we all carry due to the damage and death caused by the COVID pandemic. Even our medical experts say another round of viruses should be expected. These diseases are expensive. Secondly, countries are businesses, as mentioned in chapter 17. Businesses cannot instantaneously flip switches and change from major staple industries or philosophies and expect immediate success. There are advantages to transitional periods, and considering the amount of testing needed before a product is rolled out for sale, it can take a long time. The testing is necessary to get it right the first time. Collateral damage control from ideas that get rolled out before testing can be very expensive and usually sets these projects back even further. For example, you can't just tell all the major oil producers that they are out of business because the USA is only going to manufacture electric cars. Did anyone consider how radical environmental regulations would affect the global marketplace (stock market)? A positive example is when the EPA required a transition from the air-polluting high-sulfur diesel fuel to the new low-sulfur (cleaner burning) diesel fuels. That transition took over five years but helped clean up our air by limiting air pollutants.

Electric cars are devices to help limit air pollution, but we cannot instantaneously replace our gasoline automobiles. We do not even have a plan for the disposal of the discarded batteries. Hopefully we can return the Chinese batteries back to where they came from. Heating the interiors of electric vehicles used in America's colder climates requires very high numbers of BTUs from the electric batteries. That means those vehicles are unable to travel long distances in the winter months. The better choice is to transition from gasoline-only vehicles to more hybrid vehicles first. This gives US industries more time to invent better alternative fuel cells or even better batteries. Also, the engines in those hybrids possibly could run on a mixture of 50 percent clean-burning ethanol (grain alcohol) and gasoline. Perhaps even better, clean-burning diesel fuel. Volkswagen produced a vehicle named the Rabbit that could travel fifty miles on one gallon of diesel fuel! That may be the engine of choice for the battery-charging systems in hybrid vehicles. Thirdly, and foremost, China is our world's largest air polluter. They may sell electric car batteries, but they are the largest contributor to our world's air pollution since 2006. They pollute our air by burning coal, and continue to do so, causing anthropogenic global warming.

In an earlier chapter I mentioned that China is presently the largest manufacturer of everything. They are making all the profits from their consumers, and they should and can afford to pay for the Green New Deal, not the USA. They benefited tremendously from the COVID-19 pandemic (internet buying frenzy or the CBD illness) and should be the key player to start cleaning up our atmosphere NOW. Whatever dates were set to exempt China from cleaning up the atmosphere until 2030 is unimaginable and without logic. Waiting for China to end air pollution in 2030 is like having an idiot neighbor that keeps throwing acid on your home or automobile, and then giving them an exemption from jail time until 2030. There isn't a judge in the world that would allow that kind of behavior or grant such an exemption. They need to clean up our air now, and they can start paying for the Green New Deal now as well. Again, the USA and the rest of the world is presently not in a good economic situation because of COVID-19 pandemic costs. The USA cannot pay for any new deal now, let alone a green one. When China runs out of money to pay for cleaning up our atmosphere, the one they are heavily polluting, then the USA will also help pay to clean it up.

The amount of air-polluting particulates that leaves Asia and covers the Pacific Ocean and other parts of the world has led to the increase in temperature changes in our atmosphere, causing ocean water temperature changes, which has increased the number of cyclones in the Western Pacific Ocean. The question is, has the lower water temperature in the southern Pacific Ocean caused higher temperatures or drought conditions to western North America? I would think weather balloons that monitor these conditions may tell some nations what effect their air pollution has caused or will cause on the world's other regions. This is neither El Niño nor La Niña weather effects; these new conditions are something else. One way or another both the United States and Canada's western provinces should begin programs to prevent runaway forest fires by clear-cutting forests to produce glades. This will decrease the amount of air pollution and other environmental damage and expense they cause. Droughts can and do cause forest fires; however, 90 percent of forest fires are caused by humans. The issue is, if nations end up in world courts over air pollution, what are the documented facts in the case?

There is a lot of discussion about how we should be using our latest technologies. I believe one technology that might help two of our world's problems would be to use solar cells in an effort to desalinate Mediterranean Sea water and use it to turn the Sahara Desert into fertile land to help feed the African nations. This would benefit millions of starving people there, but also eliminate many of the hurricanes that pelt North America's eastern shorelines every year, causing devastating hardships and expenses. The Sahara desert's high heat is the cause of hurricanes that begin in the Atlantic Ocean's eastern waters.

Sometimes we can learn about our environment from movies. A 2004 sci-fi movie showed NYC and other parts of the world entering into an Ice Age when holes opened up in our upper and lower atmospheres, creating cold holes. If similar effects, such as making sure our north and south polar regions can be kept more "cloud free," it most probably would lower the temperatures there and keep the polar ice sheets from melting.

## REPURPOSING

The United States needs to lead the world in building manufacturing facilities that are able to eliminate pollutants from manufacturing processes. Furthermore, the products being produced in those facilities should be of a high quality so they can withstand refurbishing for repurposing. That should be the USA's immediate goal. It also takes energy to produce low-emission/low-polluting manufacturing technologies that would be housed in low-polluting/high-repurposing manufacturing facilities. We need to reopen the Keystone XL pipeline from Canada. At a minimum, that pipeline's oil should be dedicated to help offset energy costs for the creation of efficient high-tech, low-emission/low-pollution technologies and their facilities. That pipeline's oil is also necessary for making the asphalt to pave the roads that to go to these new facilities as well.

Instead of hiring more IRS agents to collect tax revenue, there should be an increase in EPA agents to become more astute in more modern farming methods, leading to less polluting chemicals, and also to train a new wave of manufacturers in how to produce products that are pollution-free and the benefits to making high-quality repurposed products. The EPA's new credo should be, "We no longer only regulate what we can't do (make), but train in techniques on what we can do (manufacture)!"

When I think about our health and our environment, two songs remind me of my youth and my interest in both. They are the inspiration for this chapter. They are "Nature's Way" and "Mother Nature's Son." "Nature's Way" is performed by Spirit and written by Randy California. "Mother Nature's Son" is sung by Paul McCartney and written by John Lennon and Paul McCartney. Remembering how the Cuyahoga River caught fire was definitely a significant emotional event for me. It was nature's way to motivate me to join groups to first help clean up pollutants, then prevent them.

Even though my early childhood was spent in the inner city, I had the benefit of visiting my grandfather's farm most summers. This was another significant experience for me. My sister, brother, and my cousins would often play in the barn, have to pump our water from a well, take a bath in a metal tub, and learn the idiosyncrasies of outhouse techniques. Yes, they were significant, long-lasting memories, and I very much appreciated them all.

I have mentioned that there are over four hundred national parks in the United States. If you have the opportunity to visit any one of them, I highly recommend it. Each park has its own little nuances that separates it from the others. My wife and I take many photos during our trips to the national parks we visit and look forward to visiting the ones we haven't seen. Each park has its own identifying stamp. My wife and I collect each stamp from the various parks in a stamp-collection book called a passport.

# 19.

# Education in America

When I first started writing this book in 2017, I started to notice that our country's critical values were being challenged. I said and meant *challenged* and not *changed*. Everyone in search of knowledge learns that *change is inevitable*. In 1970, my eleventh-grade social-studies teacher, Fred Schuld, played a song for our class on a record player. The song's title was "The Times They Are A-Changin'" by Bob Dylan. It was a very popular song in the early 1960s. My teacher was making the point that change is inevitable, and people should be ready for it. The United States of America has proudly been the beacon for freedom, liberties, and democracy since its founding. As we've seen through the years, greedy people and greedy nations aggressively imposed their will on the less fortunate or the unsuspecting (Pearl Harbor). Selfish people in our own country stupidly did this with slavery. The one thing missing from my teacher's point was how the selfish and powerful in our world feel they can play God and create self-fulfilling prophecies. Unfortunately, I do not believe, or at least my teacher did not teach the fact that our free nation could use the liberties entrusted to them to hate and kill the nation that was rooted in those liberties. We are all witnesses to how democracy is a fragile form of government.

In this chapter I will discuss what I have observed to be our nation's educational needs to sustain its intended founding principles and precepts and prevent its demise, being the fragile democracy that it is. This chapter discusses a base curriculum to ensure America's fundamental values. The military personnel, past and present, that fought to maintain those inherent values of liberty and freedom deserve to know that those principles *are forever*. As Abraham Lincoln said in the Gettysburg address, "These dead shall not have died in vain…and that government [democracy and the republic]…shall not perish from the earth." The Americans that created our flags, religions, and currency, and fought for democracy, were unequivocally children of emigrants. The New World, the Americas, originated as a home for people who were subjugated to oppressions, persecutions, and the threat of death. *They were not solicited to come here through false promises*, but looked for a better livelihood. Most were pressured and forced from their former homelands by the powerful and elite. Those hardworking emigrant families eventually, through God's graces, achieved a victory over their former controllers and developed a mostly peaceful "New World." It remained that way until the evils of the old world sucked Americans into two world wars. Those catastrophic events caused America to become the world's greatest interventionist. We tried to prevent future tyrants and their trademark for destruction and human suffering. The United States helped create organizations like the United Nations and the World Health Organization and others as safeguards to help preserve peace and foster human decency. Unfortunately, those created safeguards have been infiltrated by the same powerful and evil people to be used for their own devices. The United States became a strong nation because we knew for a fact and understood that evil nations preyed on the weak. Evil nations can only be held at bay by stronger nations than their own. Preventing wars and preserving peace can only be achieved through a nation's strength. Negotiations are important but not a guarantee for peace. President Ronald Reagan and many others used this phase often: "Peace through strength."

I believe that, through teaching positive historical facts about our world and our country, the United States can recover from any weakened period that ineffective leadership creates. A sound education for our children is paramount to preserve our rights and values and to sustain a strong and safe country. The United States' heritage has been to turn human suffering into hope and to be a home for peace and happiness. It should be every American's mission to maintain that heritage. America is one of the world's great wonders. However, its founding values of life, liberty, and the pursuit of happiness may conflict with any other nation's ideology or greed. Teaching about America's positive attributes, its place in the world, and that mission will foster positive attitudes for our future and its guardians: our children.

## PRESCHOOL

I have learned almost everything about preschools from my wife. She was a preschool teacher for many years and an authority in that field. To her credit, she received a national award for her efforts. When we met in college her career goal was to be an early childhood teacher. That education became invaluable as we raised our four children. From her discussions on this subject, I learned many things. For instance, preschools are organizations much like any other business. They have administrations and floor (classroom) operations. If the administration hires teachers with formal early-childhood education, the children  perform better, especially when it concerns their behavior. The administrations know they must meet state standards and requirements, housekeeping needs, and local building codes. Their marketing techniques must appease the children's busy parents, because usually they are both working full time. They know they need to develop professional and fun-filled lesson plans and programs. They also know they need an abundance of toys and creative art materials.

From my observations there is one very important requirement missing in both preschool programs and their mission statements. There isn't any mention or attention given to *respecting others' property*. Not in the sense of goods or things, but rather Thomas Paine's understanding of property as he wrote the *Rights of Man*. That is the right to life and its preservation, liberty, and property. He meant property as *our body in life*, along with what anyone acquires in their life. This fundamental principle needs to be taught right from the start to our nation's children. I know for a fact parents taught these things to their children before the 1980s boom of two working parents in every home. I have spoken often in this book about my scientific values of observation over discrimination. I have observed over the years the lack of respect by our youths for others and their property. That includes public property. There has become a selfish, twisted thought process by some who think that if they pay their tax money everything is theirs to play with. This is an important point and leads to what I call CUSP (Customary United States Principles) for the education of our American children.

Respect for other people's property should start at the preschool level and in the home by parents or legal guardians. Preschool teachers often have to instruct their classes on sharing the classroom toys. Children will often grab a toy from another classmate they are playing with. Those noble teachers need to keep order and discipline. More importantly, when they teach children about sharing, it becomes the child's first lesson on intervention. Unfortunately, unlike a family's toys or materials, all of the classroom equipment is owned by the preschool; therefore, it cannot be presented to the child in quite the same manner as if it were in the child's own home. It can be presented as the school's important materials though.

## K-8

The one thing I will always remember about my kindergarten class in the Cleveland Municipal School District was my teacher, Ms. Griffith. She played the piano and had us doing a lot of fun activities. I remember dancing in a circle with my classmates, in what appeared then to be a very large room, as she played songs. The other thing I remember was her reading many books to us. The stories were exciting and usually about adventures, like the gingerbread man. She had us using big crayons, and we always colored on manila paper. Another important detail I remember was the large amount of cardboard building blocks that were available for us to play with. I recall once we worked feverishly to build an automobile. She taught good social skills about working together to achieve a goal. The tactile experience of fitting together those large blocks was also a positive. I cannot emphasize enough how important tactile experiences are and how they need to be in our children's activities *every day*. If we keep pushing electronic pads there will not be enough time for real-world tactile necessities. The only real advantage for electronic devices is to make the few Big Tech corporations even bigger.

It is interesting that I do not recall many of my first- and second-grade experiences. I have to believe that teaching the alphabet and phonics in the first grade, then placing word associations into phrases and sentences in the second grade, must have been a very trying experience for everyone. Basic arithmetic probably wasn't much fun either. However, nothing comes from nothing, and if it weren't for the hard work put forward by those resolute teachers, I don't believe we would be living in this wonderful nation we have today. Those first- and second-grade teachers of mine were all called "colored" back then, and probably referred to as African Americans today. Whatever the politically correct want to call them, I owe them, respected them, and I will forever be indebted to them for their hard work.

My daughter teaches third grade in an urban school. I often hear about today's school lessons from her. Like my urban teachers in Cleveland, she teaches in the same manner. My teachers understood the difficult job they had. For teachers, there isn't much time for children to be fooling around and dragging their programs behind schedule. Today the principals handle the tough discipline problems. In my day, any disruptive student would be paddled. I am not saying I am in favor of corporal punishment today, only that is how it *was* handled. I am not being judgmental when I say this, but it is a fact: in a family with two parents working full time, there is a lack of discipline being taught simply because there is no time in their family's scheduled program for it. It is simple arithmetic. If you are not home with your children, how do you have the time to institute fundamental principles like discipline and respect? The elementary school teachers have to wrestle with discipline and bad behavior problems daily, more often in the public schools than the private ones. Why is this? Parents often research which schools are the best schools for their children, and many ask about discipline and expect it. The lack of discipline at the K-12 level in the public-school systems is why I am an advocate for military schools (private and government) as options. Those schools should be in *every* large urban city in America. The government should provide transportation for these students at no cost. I believe inner-city school-aged children need more discipline in their life, and military schools may provide that option. Hopefully, these schools will produce significant results. The goal is to improve urban life and the city's safety and security holistically. If adding these schools does that, then let the bells ring out.

A few years ago, I had an opportunity to be a sixth-grade substitute history teacher in a local suburban public school. I am a certified teacher in the State of Ohio, and history has always been a passion of mine. I enjoyed the times I taught at my previous organizations before my retirement. I also taught electronics at the local vocational schools in the area. It was fun to be working with kids and taking them through American and world history. My experiences taught me an important observation. I call it the one-in-ten rule: For every ten students you have in your class, one student will be disruptive . If you have twenty students, the class will have two dissidents, and so on.

One day, our class was reviewing the next day's test. I noticed that one of the students was preoccupied with a different textbook than our history book. When I went up to his desk, he quickly closed the book. I asked him what was so interesting in the book. I opened it and found that he had hollowed out the center section of pages and was playing a handheld-sized electronic game in it. I took him to the principal's office to let the administration handle the situation. My biggest problem with what he had done was not that the boy was playing a game instead of reviewing for a test with us, but the fact that he had destroyed a textbook. It was the school's property, taxpayers' property, and that was the most upsetting thing to me. Through years of teaching I would have others challenge me in my class activities, but I learned to expect some bad behavior. However, once they abuse any public or private property, that is another matter. It is destructive and counterproductive and shows a lack of respect for all people.

## HIGH SCHOOL

For many of this book's chapters I have done tons of research. I reviewed subjects like drug abuse, garbage collection, or how many people voted for whoever. I'm not going to do that research for this section on high-school education. There is plenty of data out there about graduation numbers, what students are doing in state schools, public or private, dropout numbers, or ratios between inner-city students and suburban. All this data is available on the internet, and I hope you review it, because information about high-school students is information about our country's future.

What I am going to talk about in this section is something I know about high schools through my own experiences. I know it sounds like an "I want to talk about me" thing. However, if I did not think it was an important aspect for this section's intent, I wound have left out my personal experience.

When I started high school in ninth grade at Independence High School in Independence, Ohio, I did not know what to expect, even though both my older brother and sister attended that same school. I knew I would be playing football and other sports and that I was not college-bound. I just went day to day with no goals. I took in all the social aspects of high school though, like gaining friendships, learning to drive a car, going to Friday or Saturday night dances, and all the other things ninth and tenth graders did. When it came to schoolwork, it seemed that most of the teachers who tried to push me to study found a tough kid who pushed back. I suppose the administration and the teachers had enough to worry about with the Vietnam War going on. These teachers and administrators never knew from day to day when they would have to make another morning public announcement about a recent graduate who was killed in the war. Therefore, trying to deal with a few bullheaded kids wasn't a priority for them. The schools' attitude was probably like professional coaches and managers when a star player is in a contract holdout. When asked by the media about that player being out of training camp for whatever reason, the pat answer is, "I have enough to worry about with the players that are here working their butts off than to worry about the ones that aren't here." So, I just basically skated along those first two years.

It was in the summer of 1969 when my education took a bad turn. That summer many of my close friends decided to quit school. There were sixteen out of about four hundred students that did quit. For a suburban school back then that was a high number of dropouts. The constant pressure I put on my two hardworking parents for me to quit school finally paid off. They reluctantly gave up and let me quit high school. There was one condition though: I had to find a full-time job, and I did. It was a 7:00 a.m., to 4:00 p.m. union-paid grocery store clerk position. I happily did that job, lived at home, and my relationship with my parents was better than ever. That whole winter of 1969 and spring of 1970 was all about routine, and I became part of what the hippies of the day would call "the establishment." Yes, a seventeen-year-old kid entered into adulthood.

A very serious event happened to me that May in 1970 (and to Kent State with a tragedy). The part-time high school seniors that I worked with at the grocery store were all celebrating the fact that they graduated from high school. I worked with many of these kids. I saw them making the grade on one hand and taking the next step on the other. I felt I could never achieve their level of happiness. I began to think that I was being passed up by the others and felt like less of a person.

If anybody knows anything about me though, they will tell you that I never back down from a challenge. I came home that evening and told my mother and father that I had decided to go back and graduate from high school. I told them that I not only wanted to graduate, but to do so with my original classmates as it was intended.

A day or two later I met with my high-school guidance counselor and told him of my plan. Fortunately, I had completed most of my require-ments for ninth and tenth grade, except for my tenth-grade English course. The most difficult part was to complete two years of high school in one year. My counselor formulated a plan and laid it out for me and my parents. This was at a time when the GED (general equivalency diploma) and internet classes did not exist. I would have to physically go through summer school for two classes. That was unfortunate for me because it took me off my school's football team.

I took tenth-grade English and algebra in summer classes at a Cleveland public school and did fairly well. During the regular school year I did not have any study halls or breaks. I had to take both my eleventh-and twelfth-grade social studies and English classes. I also had to take night-school classes. They were psychology and current events. The most interesting thing about all the class work was that *I welcomed it.* In the end I graduated with my class and earned the parent teacher association scholarship. I decided to attend Kent State University in the fall.

Besides receiving the PTA scholarship, the other award I received was the Veterans of Foreign Wars' Voice of Democracy Award. The VFW award theme that year was to write on the topic "Was Manifest Destiny America's Destiny?"

I remember my mother trying to help me write this paper. I had to give her credit since she only completed the eleventh grade. However, history, especially American history, was always my strong suit. I was destined to win on a subject about America's destiny. So in the end, I had a wonderful high school experience.

People can learn a lot from old movies about history and public schools. I recently watched the 1955 movie *Blackboard Jungle*, starring Glen Ford and Sydney Portier. This movie was about teaching in New York City's public high schools in the early 1950s. This correlates with what is happening in our nation's public schools today. The challenge for those teachers back then was that they were trying to teach in an era when young adults were only raised by working mothers because their fathers had gone off to fight in either WWII or the Korean War. The mothers of those children tried to juggle finding work and living without the companionship of a male influence in their family. The movie told how it was impossible to instill any discipline in the homes of adolescent children in the single-parent households.

## COLLEGE

My thoughts about a K-12 education, college, and beyond are that you can't learn without seeing what is at the end of the rainbow. The rainbow for American children or any children should lead to successful careers and, more importantly, an abundance of high-paying jobs here in the United States. I said in the chapter on family that our parents wanted to build a better America than the one they had. My parents grew up during the Great Depression. So, for them, anything they built was better than the ground zero they had to live in. As a parent of four children, I tried to build a better situation in America than what I had. I believe my children are trying to do that for their children. In that building process there has to be a vision of the rainbow, and you must follow it until you find that pot o' gold at its end. The pot of gold could be as simple as a job washing windows, but that is your personal pot of gold. Whatever your goals are, know there are people and support groups available for you. If you do not have parents or friends, various groups are available to help you achieve your goals. A great online job tool is LinkedIn. A non-online group is every state's unemployment office. The biggest roadblock keeping you from achieving your goals may be YOU.

I believe the biggest issue and problem in America today is college debt. It is a killer because the United States lacks their former manufacturing industries, which provided higher wages. This problem has forced high school students to seek higher-paid jobs hopefully through higher education. Basically the two problems are tied together. Both deleting higher-paying union-wage jobs and increasing college enrollment, which really has become a supply/demand, cause/effect problem. If a nation transitions from a manufacturing base, like the United States was until the 1990s, and goes into a service-based economy, this is a problem. The EPA mandates did not help and still do not help with this problem. They should be informing the industries and other businesses in America what they can safely manufacture instead of telling them what they cannot manufacture.

The manufacturing jobs paid very well for many years, more than service-type (restaurant) jobs. Due to the lack of these higher-paying jobs, high school students by necessity were herded into colleges and universities at the thought of achieving higher-paying jobs. Had the manufacturing jobs remained, they would still be providing higher union-scale wages as an option for young Americans. I believe if that discussed transition had not happened, we would not be in the college debt crisis we are in. Our own EPA's rigid requirements for manufacturing businesses did not and still does not help.

The higher-learning institutions are no different than any other industries or businesses. They too fall under the simple system of supply and demand and lower interest rates from which to borrow on. When the demand increases and the industry doesn't have the capability or capacity to supply it, the prices get raised naturally, in some cases to deter the increase in demand. Our national and state governments then and today see the increase in unemployment or underemployment and give grants to colleges to offset their business costs. What I described is a fact in our history and simple economics. Whenever the government interferes in any industry to "fix it," they always create other problems because of interfering with the natural laws of supply and demand. The states pumped money into their state schools to also help colleges with their bombardment of students, and of course, maintain their all-important football and basketball programs. The problem was and is, where are the jobs for these college graduates? The federal government ended up in the student loan business. They gave colleges money on the one hand to help them stay economically (and socially) solvent, and went into the loan (shark) business on the other hand. What should have been created is a stimulus for newer, cleaner, more energy-efficient manufacturing plants and the jobs that would follow. A policy to BUY MADE IN AMERICA would have been a no-brainer for everyone to invest in. Buying many foreign-made products instead of our own only adds to the college-debt problem. College graduates need to understand another reason why their costs have skyrocketed and caused higher loans: It is because they have been paying for loan costs but also the cost associated for "free-riding" students, foreign and native students that claim to be disadvantaged. That process has caused higher student-loan costs, and the disadvantaged claims need to be capped.

## THE SCHOOL OF HARD KNOCKS

There is an old saying that there is no substitute for experience. Truer words were never spoken. There is an offshoot to this style of learning that almost never receives any praise, and that is learning through the school of "hard knocks." Not many people want to admit they were fooled. I suppose hard knocks could be classified as an intangible. However, it usually produces significant learning through painful experiences. We all have or should have had some formal education to prepare us in life. However, life was never meant to be a feel-good ride without any bumps.

I really believe that God's plan is to be our protector. God is there for you in the long run of life. God wants you to make the right decisions. Only you can choose the right decisions with your experience and weigh the good with the bad to help with those decisions. When I think of hard knocks, it reminds me of the musical *Annie*. The movie's star, Annie (of the once famous comic strip *Little Orphan Annie*), sings the song, "It's the Hard Knock Life." It is a hard-knocks life because of the world's uncertainties. The United States has made mistakes over the years. Americans understand and should know for a fact that they live in a democracy and have the ability to mend its mistakes. We strive to make our country better, not just for some immediate gratification but for the future, our children, and their livelihood.

## CONCLUSION

The discussions in this chapter are not about color or gender issues, but specifically about the message to stay in school and get good grades. A person's grades in their education, their experience, and their choice of a career should be the major factors in how people get placed into jobs. Students need to know unequivocally the solid standards used by business, industry, and government to evaluate them for employment. The top standard must be the grades that they obtained while in school. That standard and its emphasis should never change, or it would make a mockery of our whole educational process.

We all need to work together to make our children feel that they are in school because we believe they can have a positive effect on their future and America's future. An important part of this equation is to sustain higher-paying employment in the manufacturing industries in America for those that do not or should not go to college (debt). Instead of hiring 85,000 more IRS agents to ensure that our politicians get their paycheck, we should be hiring more EPA staff, not to prevent American manufacturing but rather redirect Americans on how to manufacture safe, non-polluting products and supply-chain technologies. It was and will always be in America's best interest to maintain a solid manufacturing base to provide higher wages over lower-paying service industry jobs and to maintain our great middle class. Increasing American manufacturing will help in keeping our nation strong and safe from our adversaries.

The music that inspired me to write this chapter came from the songs "The Times They Are A-Changin'," sung and written by Bob Dylan, and "Another Brick in the Wall," performed by Pink Floyd and sung by Roger Waters. Bob Dylan says in this song that our children do not listen to their parents anymore. He hit that one right on the head. Our children should learn and understand that their parents are trying to build security nests for their families, called their homes. They are not trying to stifle their social growth, only to assure that they live safely enough to be able to have their children also live in a safe environment. I'm all for the schools that seem like they are overprotecting our children with building security, as well. It makes children feel like their parents have placed them into an environment that may be even safer than their own homes. That should be a good start to every child's day.

The message I receive when I hear the song "Another Brick in the Wall" is the story of the Three Bears—the homes of straw, sticks, and bricks. My take on that is, "Hey teachers, keep reading those fairy tales!" Someday the kids might just understand the fact that building strong foundations are the important things in life.

# 20.

# American Music: Our Legacy and Destiny

Music scholars believe the greatest contribution to our American music was formed from the assimilation of the many ethnic groups that fought in the American Civil War. That can be said for both the North and the South. In the evening hours, the troops would gather around their camps' evening fires and play, sing, and share their familiar songs and melodies. However, this was after Columbus discovered the Americas, and the settlements of St. Augustine, Jamestown, and Plymouth. All these events eventually led to America being the melting pot for all the world's immigrants. Make no mistake, it is that "melting pot" which has made our American music unique among all the other music in the world. The driving force behind much of that music was the newly freed slaves' excitement and jubilation due to new opportunities for love, birth, and nourishment, and the confidence in newfound freedom from the oppressions of the past. African slaves had the oppression of slavery, but they also were able to feel the joy of emancipation and the hope for a better life. There were no more chains, whips, and overseers. Our music always displayed our emotions, and our emotions were expressed in our music, songs, and the dancing that followed from those emotions.

I would be remiss if I did not tell you about the music of our indigenous American people. Some 1,500 different tribes of the Americas had certain similarities. Their instruments were mostly drums, rattles, pipes, horns, strings, and wooden sticks. The drums were made out of wood. They could be as large as a kettle, or single- or double-headed drums.

Some had coverings of animal skins. The rattles were made out of dry gourds or turtle shells. The pipes were made out of hollowed branches or dried reeds. The horns were often made from animals. The stringed instruments were attached to bows and plucked.

Our Native American music often started out slow, with a steady beat increasing in tempo and volume over time. The singers often sang along with the tempo using words, meaningless syllables, or imitating the sounds from their wild surroundings. Many of their songs were meant for special occasions, like planting and harvest times, powwows, courtships, or rituals such as their tribes' anthems. This is a generalization; however, there were many tribes, living in climates from the Artic Circle to the jungles of the Amazon. Not all had the natural materials to make the musical instruments described above. No matter the instruments, as the Americas grew through immigration the music began to morph into our own American music and will always be different than any other in the world.

The music brought to colonial New England was different than the music of our South. The New Englanders may have eventually danced to minuets, waltzes, and polkas, but their original music was based on religious psalms. As the South began to be settled, through the Appalachian Mountains many Europeans brought along country blues, fiddling, and folk music. As African slaves arrived, they brought banjos, drums, and xylophones. Later the South had an influx of Scotch-Irish, and they brought their ballads with them. In Louisiana, the French Creole and African people created the basis for Dixieland jazz. When our nation's people grew and moved westward, country-western music emerged.

When the Civil War did occur, those young soldiers were already familiar with their brand of music. Even after fighting through some of the bloodiest battles the world had ever seen, those young, mostly pale-faced men would play their music. When you average *three hundred deaths per day*—that was the toll for just the Northern troops—it can get very ugly for humans to witness. They played their music to remind themselves of why they were fighting, *to end slavery*, and to remember the joyful times in their lives and their promise to bring peace once again to the land.

Below is a chart showing the music that developed in America from its beginning. Much of the music styles listed overlap in time, because Americans have always liked a variety of music and have always been open to new styles. Americans listened to these new styles and began to feel the musicians' message and how they felt through their music. One thing is for certain though: What has made our American music different is what makes our music better. See figure 20-A for a review of our music's history.

| Type of Music | Time Period | Instruments | Associated Dancing |
|---|---|---|---|
| Indigenous | 8000 BC to present | Drums, Rattles, Pipes, Horns, Sticks | Stomp or Traditional to each Tribe |
| Religious Hymns (Psalms) | 1600s | Organ Music (as they arrived) | None |
| Classical-German, French | 1700s | Orchestra Ensemble | Waltz & Minuet |
| Gospel (various offshoots) | Late 1700s | Vocals, Low Instrumentation | None |
| Polka - Czech and Polish | Early 1800s | Orchestra Ensemble | Polka, Waltz |
| Hillbilly (Appalachian) | Late 1700s – Early 1800s | Fiddles, Guitars, Banjos, Jugs, Drums | Dance to the Fiddlers, Promenade |
| Folk | Early 1800s | Fiddles, Guitars, Banjos, Jugs, Drums | Square, Barn, Reel, Jig, various akin to their native lands |

| | | | |
|---|---|---|---|
| Western (Country) | Mid-1800s | Harmonica, Guitar, Fiddle | Line Dance, Two-step |
| Blues | Late 1800s | Piano, Guitar, Organ, Harmonica, Bass Fiddle | Slow Dancing |
| Ragtime | Around 1900 | Mainly Piano | Turkey Trot, Old Barn Dance |
| Dixieland | Early 1900s | Trumpets, Trombones, Saxophones, Clarinets, Percussion | Cajun Jig, The Charleston |
| Bluegrass | Early 1900s | Vocals, Many String Instruments | Clogging |
| Hawaiian | 1910s | Ukulele, Xaphoon, Ka'eke'eke, Ipe, Pahu | Hula Kahiko (ancient) and Hula 'Auana (modern) |
| Modern Country | 1920s | Guitar, Fiddle, Small Band Ensemble | Two-Step, Polka, Promenade, Waltz |
| Swing (Jazz) | 1930s | Solo Artist with Big Bands | Jitterbug, Lindy Hop |
| Rhythm & Blues | 1940s | Piano, Trumpet, Saxophone, Drums, Small Bands | Jitterbug, Lindy Hop |
| Doo-Wop | Late 1940's | Vocals, Low Instrumentation | Slow dance |
| Rock and Roll | Early 1950s | Piano, Saxophone, Guitar, Drums, Small Bands | The Twist, Swim, Mashed Potato |
| Funk | Mid-1950s | Electric Guitar and Bass, Keyboard, Drum | Popping and Locking |

| Soul | Mid-1950s | Vocals, Electric Guitar, Bass, Keyboard, Drum, Percussion | Northern Soul |
|------|-----------|-----------------------------------------------------------|---------------|
| Surf | Early 1960s | Electric Guitar and Bass, Keyboard, Drum | Surfer Stomp |
| Tejano | Early 1950s | Accordion, Guitar, Bajo Sexto, Brass, Drum, Flute | Mambo, Bolero, Polka, Waltz |
| Motown Style | Early 1960s | Vocals, Electric Guitar, Bass, Tambourine, Drum | Swing Style |
| Hard Rock | Mid-1960s | Electric Guitar, Electric Bass, Drums, Vibrato | Moshing |
| Punk | Mid-1970s | Vocals, Electric Guitar and Bass, Drum | Pogo |
| Disco | Early 1970s | Horns, Electric Piano, Rhyme Guitars, Synthesizer | Disco |
| Salsa | Early 1970s | Conga Drums, Maracas, Claves, Bass, Flute | Salsa |
| Reggae | Mid-1960s | Electric Guitar and Bass, Keyboard, Drums | Bogle |
| Hip-Hop | Mid-1970s | Drum Machines, Keyboard, Piano, Turntable, Sampler | Hip Hop |
| Rap Hip-Hop | Mid-1980s | Drum Machines, Keyboard, Piano, Turntable, Sampler | Hip Hop |

| Modern Tejano | Early 1980s | Accordion, Guitar, Bajo Sexto, Electric Bass, Drum, Synthesizer, Flute, Violin | Mambo, Bolero, Polka, Waltz |
|---|---|---|---|

Figure 20-A

The songs that inspired me to write this chapter were "Rock and Roll Heaven" and "American Pie." "Rock and Roll Heaven" was performed by the Righteous Brothers and written by Johnny Stevenson and Alan O'Day. "American Pie" was written and performed by Don McLean.

Our American music is about the musicians who wrote songs for people so they could *connect* with them. It was a communication tool before people ever thought of it being a communication tool. Their audience loved to hear it, play it, and dance to it. Those musicians had stories to tell and built them into those songs. The Righteous Brothers and Don McLean hit their bullseyes with their two songs. For Don McLean, "American Pie" was considered the fifth best song of the twentieth century by RIAA (Recording Industry Association of America) in their project *Songs of the Century.*

The Righteous Brothers sang about the many rock 'n' roll artists who died prematurely in the late twentieth century. The first musician was Jimi Hendrix. Hendrix, as he was called by my friends and I, was one of my all-time favorite musicians. I was saddened by his death. However, all the artists that are mentioned in the song "Rock and Roll Heaven" greatly contributed to our American musical heritage. I believe as they sang in this song that every one of us is a star, just as the many stars paint pictures in the dark of night. God has made everyone special to shine in their own way. Each of us has our own song to sing. If you become so blessed to go to heaven, there are a lot of bands and musicians up there to listen to.

Don McLean in interviews has said how much the rock 'n' roll period affected his life. In singing "American Pie" he is giving a tribute to the early years of rock 'n' roll and how he lived through them. I believe our American music helped make our moral soul, and it can *save our American soul.* I believe our music can help raise our spirits to have America once again be the beacon for world peace and help riddle out the hate. It was Marvin Gaye who sang in his song "What's Goin' On," that "only love can conquer hate." In Don McLean's song he touches on his love for slow dancing. He made a great point with that. Slow dancing is a good step in the right direction for couples, simply as their wedding dance.

These two songs affected me because I believe that I am a religious person and believe in heaven and life thereafter. People today are rushing around trying to get 144 years of life's pleasures in about their normal seventy-two-year life span. Why? I believe more and more people have lost their faith and have turned their back on God. I believe people need to take in life as it comes to them in every moment each day. In professional football they say the greatest quarterbacks have success when they let the pace of the game come to them. It is when every play seems to slow down, and then they can react to it. The successful, experienced quarterbacks know this. They may have five different receivers to throw to on any pass play. However, they know the one player that they practiced with the most, and who is the one not being covered by the defense. That experience allows them the "vision" to most likely make a successful play. It wasn't the coach who designed the play, or the fans in the stands that want a certain play, or the many Monday-morning quarterbacks who complain about some plays. Why can't most people be like the successful quarterbacks and know how to run their own life? That is, to let things come to them, as they have learned in their life, naturally, instead of rolling the dice and going only for the gusto. Better yet, living the life that the internet and our entertainment industry is trying to push everybody into. Try to live with no cellphones, no advertisements, no internet, and no bad news every morning.

My wife always says, "It is a great day to have a great day." It is so true. You can control having a good or bad day. It starts with your attitude. In the chapter on religion I mentioned Zoroastrianism. Its main principle is that there is good and evil in all humans. They believe that the evil that is in all of us has to be suppressed every day. Their simple math is that by practicing removing the evil, only the good will remain. Many of the worlds' religions tell us the same thing. One prayer is, "lead us not into temptation but deliver us from evil." With all those great teachings, I'm ready to hear some "good for the soul" gospel music. So let's imagine for a moment and hear that singing, clapping, movin' and a-groovin', and thank God for this great day and the wonderful people in it!

Make no mistake: I love America and I love all Americans, even though some may lose sight of the important things in life. In the end, it is important for all of us to understand that we are all in this together. Not any one of us is greater or more important than the other. I've said many times in this book that envy and egos are dangerous things. Try practicing what my wife says about every day being a great day to have a great day. Start listening to more music and less bad news. Reflect on each of your day's activities every night. My wife recently told me that her father said his evening prayers every night. He was a great person with a lot of faith. Incidentally, he and Elvis Presley were born in the same year. I bet they both had many fond rock 'n' roll memories and the singing and dancing that went with each song.

I am not naïve; I know that many people are suffering in our world. I know things may seem pretty tough at times, and maybe you feel your life is a waste or has been wasted. There is no better feeling though when people join organizations that help people who *really* need help, even more than you think you do. After visiting and helping these people, many people begin to realize that their life really has a purpose. I believe yours does. If you choose the right paths, those paths can make you happy. I am hopeful that someday you may start whistling to some music's tune. Doing that simple act is continuing our American music's legacy and its destiny.

# 21.

# A New Age for Reasoning

I hope you have found this book to be both entertaining and enlightening. As much fun as I had writing this book, there were four chapters that were very difficult to write and not much fun at all. Those chapters were the prologue (due to discussing the world-changing COVID-19 pandemic), the one on various media, the divorce chapter, and this one. As difficult as it was for me to write them, this book would have been hollowed of its main purpose; that is to be more observant to our nation's important issues and to help the *legitimately* needy people.

For the last twenty-five years or so, I have noticed that people have been ignoring many important issues facing our nation's future, our children's future. In this book's preface I labelled the twenty-first century as "the century of self-fulfilling prophecies." For the very rich people and powerful nations this century has become like a plaything to feed their selfish actualization needs, disregarding others or humanity itself. After discussing these important observed issues about the United States and what I call Greater America (North and South America), I knew trying to convince people to take more time to evaluate important events and even their very own soul would be a tough sell. For instance, our large media outlets have made conclusions about national events by finger-pointing in the *opposite direction* instead of more plausible explanations. In 2022, the polling service's numbers showed that our nation was more politically divided than in prior years. It could be because of the media's reverse logic on reporting events or purposely not reporting them, specifically the political stories. This led to increasing the USA's political dissension and widened the gap already created, mostly by the media since the 2016 presidential election. The large media outlets and our entertainment industry must have been overjoyed knowing that the data showed that their political coverage and the dividing of our people verified that they officially became "the tail wagging the dog." You, as the paying TV audience and customer, are the dog that should wag its tail, and they made themselves the tail, wagging you, the dog. Their listeners, due to the pandemic, became hooked on their updates instead of switching to watching old movies, listening to music, or even, heaven forbid, reading books. Chalk up another victory for large corporations and one more loss for the consumers. Today in 2024, we might ask ourselves, where is the promise from the 2020 Democratic National Convention for an increase in cooperation among us for a more loving and respectful society? People *who take the time* to notice our society's further division are asking themselves, why is this happening?

In murder cases, investigators look for the *logic and reasons* for their cases. They look for the motives, means, opportunities, and especially the process of *following the money trail* to find the culprits. With the advent and use of artificial intelligence, we can add following the data (information) or non-information trail (not reported) to find possible causes. A mentor of mine once told me, "information is power." Perhaps that is why the Big Tech corporations, large TV news networks, and possibly our government squash or twist information. Recent events like pandemics released just prior to a presidential election, as in 2020, or the national budget buster it caused, are events to be scrutinized as to why they happened. You may add the invasion across our borders and the increase of seemingly endless news coverage of racial tensions. This all cannot be by chance or coincidence. There is too much at stake for some of the highly organized and powerful groups. The fact is, the TV networks and their advertisers are making too much money on increasing the USA's division, because it has captured a profitable audience for them. Many believe the large TV-network owners are having their employees use what is called the "double drop" method. That is when they are paid to advertise products on air, but also paid not to report on certain news, because some very rich and powerful people do not want certain news stories broadcast because they do not support their political ideology. WE NEED MORE NEWS CONDUITS.

In my life I have been fortunate to work in many different fields: as a livery stable hand, in grocery and department retail stores, warehousing, shipping and receiving, purchasing, electrical and electronic repair and design, teaching, technical writing, project management, and quality assurance. It is a wide spectrum. I've seen a lot from a technical point of view, but also the humanitarian side. What is happening in the United States, the dysfunction and periodic chaos, is happening by a purposeful, designed cartel of the world's largest network of technical corporations (called Big Tech), their trading partners, and powerful politicians. That described group has also become a cartel for most of the information channels we use every day, and it has become dangerously destructive. An important point to considered is that they hold the reins of artificial intelligence. I've heard these groups use soft words like *transformation*, but for the people trying to deal with the hardships of everyday life it is called *evil*. Yes, a transformation is happening, but by design of the internet controllers, television and entertainment industries, and their business partnerships. However, any transformation in the USA should be made by us, the paying-for-products customers who use these devices, and the largely tax-paying citizenry. We are the people who mostly pray for peace and unity and not divisiveness. We had better do something about this transformation soon, because if we don't, there will not be anything left to transition to.

For us, the middle class, we are being targeted because we are an economic threat. We labor to earn wages from mostly sincere sources and try to limit government's leeching attempt at our personal growth. As our families attempt to build equity, government takes it away by increasing our taxes or limiting energy sources, which raises production costs and equates to price increases. It has been the goal of that cartel to squeeze the life out of our earned wages. The cartels' actions are the complete reversal of making America glorious. By continually squeezing our earnings they are taking our historic and prosperous middle class down. Our great middle class is what made America the greatest country in the world.

I do not get any pleasure out of saying this, but there is an evil trend developing today by this aforementioned cartel of enterprises and their partnerships. I believe we are presently in some kind of war. It is not a Cold War as it once was between the USA and the USSR and Red China, or a hot war like with the many Middle East nations. There is an insane amount of international money being thrown around like confetti. I believe we are in a "gold war," or a money war, and the information channels we all use is their COVED intelligence to win this war. For this cartel it becomes more profitable for them if we, the middle class, do not spend our money to build any equity, but to live in a system as renters and never own anything that holds any value. Perhaps these cartels are looking to expand (investing) in apartment living (renting) and sour on anything that resembles home ownership and the equity that may come with that. If the American dream is for home ownership, there are going to be some very angry immigrants who have been crossing our borders since 2021. We know this because a minimum wage offers only subsistence and creates the necessity for renting instead of owning anything that holds any value. This minimum wage push has been a factual trend in our country for over the last two decades. It has become more and more difficult for us to afford to pay for things like car leases and housing rent while working two jobs.

In earlier chapters I discussed the need to not judge too quickly on issues or events until as much information or data as possible can be collected. However, the problem is *and will always be that it takes time* to do so. Earlier I referenced what is called English logic. That is the process of gathering information, making decisions from a few choices, then acting. In some cold-case murder investigations it can take many years to get the evidence to make an arrest and conviction. Unfortunately, what are the portals for information being used by our brains today to make logical conclusions as to what is happening to our nation's economy or government? We have to face the realities that most of our information is being transmitted to us by our various media sources using the popularized hi-tech, pocket-sized gadgetry that we carry with us today. They are our little brainwashing devices called smartphones. These devices are very intelligent for *their* makers. However, they no longer are mostly used as telephones. The naïve people using them are missing a very important fact. These devices are not only output, but also dangerous input devices. The data being transmitted by the device makers is being gathered to get the reactionary (in most cases the emotional) responses from their monitored subjects. This is problematic. The fact is the second largest producer of these devices is our nation's largest monetary adversary, the PRC, or Communist China. As users we are not following what our Fifth Amendment to the US Constitution calls "the right to remain silent." We are foolishly giving up the right to privacy and our personal business. Every button on that little device is sending information (data) about you to Big Tech or its partners to give to any bidder. The data is not verbal, but because it is keystroked, it is tracked as written. Maybe that's why there is the big push today to eliminate telephone customer services (because it is verbal) and have everyone go to a written chat. You almost never discuss your question with a knowledgeable person. A "chat" is an oxymoron because it isn't a verbal chat (conversation) at all. Welcome to the new age of pigeonholing telecommunication help lines that only further frustrate an already dysfunctional society. The fact is that all of our computers, especially the smartphones, are "cells," a tentacle or arm for controlling use by artificial intelligence.

Our former means of getting information from newspapers, by word of mouth, our friends, families, other associations, and even the local yellow pages, are used less and less because they are purposely being made more unavailable. Again, this of course is being done by design and not just some trendy cost-cutting thing. This increase of the habitual use of these electronic devices became more evident when the COVID-19 pandemic occurred. More and more people were locked down into their dwellings and relied heavily on their electronic devices for updates on the medical side of the pandemic, unemployment benefits, and new employment opportunities.

I believe the worst-case scenario relative to information channels is when the vital information is not being dispersed. Hence *there is a purpose for needing a new age of reasoning by everyone.* However, how can anyone clearly reason things out if the information we need is either held back or lies? We depend on facts to make wise decisions. I used the word *lies* because there is a growing trend, and it's seemingly acceptable today, for a certain political ideology to use lying to achieve their mission to control the world. To put it plainly, "we the people...in order to form a more perfect union [one without discord], establish justice, insure domestic tranquility, provide for the common defense, promote the general welfare, and secure the blessings of liberty" *need true factual information.* A move to socialism, which uses any means to justify its end purposes to control the world, uses lying to conceal facts from those seeking truth.

With the recent economic turmoil cast on everyone in this post-pandemic period, it has led to some hot stories out there for the newsies. So much so, they could easily spend twenty-four hours a day covering them. However, what has been rightly news is not being investigated nor mentioned by our largest media outlets. If I were a professional news reporter or journalist and I had a "hot" story, and after it was edited for fact-finding and legal opinion and it was rejected for publication, I would want to know why. If it was given the usual "corporate says so," I believe a whistleblower protection law, federal shield law, or the journalists' or writers' own guilds or unions should protect them and their stories. Unilaterally, there also needs to be legal protection to the news agencies or media from any actions as a result of releasing news stories until all the facts are heard.

Another limiting factor of our freedom of information is the fact that the internet *is* a monopolized information conduit. I say monopoly because there is only *one* internet. It is like having one television channel, or one radio station. It does not have any competition from other cyber portals such as something that may be called the "ultranet" or "govnet" or "publicnet" or, even better, "Iam4localbiznet" (I American are for local business network). We all have witnessed over the past thirty years how the internet can easily be sickened with viruses and hacked. Providing anything to everyone has been more of an expensive problem for most people than a solution. Even the word *cyberspace* itself is another one of those new purposeful reversals like the word *chat*. One would envision *cyberspace* to be an infinite space that anyone at any time can travel to. The fact is, it is a single channel or conduit from its inception as an Ethernet cable, is not totally open to anyone, and only uses one language: binary. We need more channels from which to receive information, and those channels must be more clinical and less volatile. Even our older technology of radio and television had an array of frequencies as alternatives, which allowed for competition and growth within that technology. The internet has so many problems from not being flawless or secure I believe if the present internet had competing "nets" with newer technologies and methods built in for consumer protection, present internet users would switch from using it.

The Big Tech makers of these devices and their programs which allow internet access have everyone lining up to use them. Unfortunately, we have become so emotionally and habitually attached to these devices, like smartphones, it's almost as though *you can't help yourself* without their use. The use and transfer of purposeful messages by Big Tech's TV advertising partners causes a funneling or corralling effect whereby they have you hooked. This monopolized conduit's design is similar to having cattle funneled into corrals for slaughter. Big Tech's conduit produces and creates for their business partnerships with app vendors with no optional clauses for site visitors and required cookie usage with those vendor partners. Basically, internet users are finding that if you refuse to accept cookies or the app, you will not get the information you may require. Using QR codes only increases their control over everyone and endangers every user's monetary privacy. They force users to go to one of their few stores to get the website's full access. I don't know what millennials and Gen Z call it, but my generation called that blackmail. If you do not believe that Big Tech and their partners know you are hooked, why do you think that almost every TV commercial in 2023 and 2024 shows a picture of a smartphone? They know you are attached to it, and when you see the commercial you will habitually look for it, pick it up, and use it. You may not remember, but visuals of smartphones were not used as often before 2023.

As a nation of compassionate people, please take more time to reason out why the information you receive today may be being used against our nation's world positioning or our democracy itself and trying to influence you. Gather your information, scrutinize it, make your decisions, and then act. However, that information must be factual. It is so important to get factual information. The most important reason is that it is needed for important issues, perhaps as simple as a political candidate's position on issues.

Your vote is your vote and your decision. The question remains: Who or what is supplying the information for your decisions? How people voted in the 2020 elections spoke volumes about where the American middle class is at today: poorer. As stated in chapter 17 about government, *governments are businesses too*. Without sound fiscal policies, the United States could become just another broken down third-world nation. The global information cartel discussed is a powerful and influential controlling force on our decision-making today. This being a voting democracy, we need to reverse the trend of allowing a malfunctioning internet to have anything to do with our voting machinery. As mentioned, there is too much money at stake for the controlling Big Tech cartel for them to not put their fingers on the scales and use the internet to cause election chaos. Only the use of closed-circuit or other secure transfers of information should be used relative to our democratic voting systems to make it more secure, but *absolutely no voting* data should be transmitted over the internet. Know that when the information cartel controls the media and the internet, they are controlling your thought processes with every colorful picture on your LCD screens and every keystroke. It is not much different than if you were wearing one of those virtual reality helmets. The visions being displayed are taking you for a ride down the information cartel's designed game of controlling your thoughts and then your decisions.

Before the USA's entry into World War II, the continued aerial bombardment by Nazi Germany was Great Britain's darkest hour. Britain's Prime Minister Winston Churchill told his people to "Never, never, never give up" to the enemy forces. Today, freedom-loving people must never, never, never give up to the information controllers of the day, or we will be nothing but slaves to them. We cannot allow ourselves to be electronically funneled or corralled and pinned down by them. Our biggest and most important ammunition against powerful groups is to keep the sovereignty of our voting process and to regulate the evil selfishness of those controlling forces. As mentioned, the internet is not a secure   conduit. It has flaws. We can never allow any tabulated votes to travel into the *trail of the highwaymen* relative to the sovereignty of our voting system. It is critical that alternative methods for transferring voting data should be made through more secure conduits as mentioned earlier, such as closed-circuit lines or other methods.

## THE NEED FOR A SECOND POLITICAL
## PARADIGM SHIFT IN FOUR YEARS

In chapter 17 we discussed a few subject matters, one being politics. I mentioned that my first experience with politics was the 1960 presidential race when I was only seven years old. I did not mention that my middle-class family members were dedicated voting Democrats. My father was a steelworker and my mother was a meatcutter and later an aerospace worker. My mother's father and her three brothers were all steelworkers. As an aerospace worker, my mother was also a union steward in the International Association of Machinists and Aerospace Workers. I cannot say for sure why my parents had the political convictions they had, but in their time they, like many others, understood that the best way for the middle class to increase their income was to organize and bargain for sharing in an organization's monetary growth. If a large industry or corporation had growth (I emphasize *large* and *had growth*), the workers in the operation deserve to receive earnings commensurate with that growth. Most people working in a large for-profit organization feel that way. The point is that the American labor force has been supporting Democratic candidates for many years because they felt it gave them the best opportunity for personal growth.

I believe the unionized American middle class must be confused and disillusioned by their leadership's position on many of the political issues and the candidates that they have supported in recent years. If their leadership supports anything other than an individual's financial growth, it clearly has failed in its representation. I'm sure many in our unions' leadership positions and prospective politicians are asking themselves the same question. Before the 2020 presidential election, the Democratic Party supported a drastic increase to the minimum wage. My point here is that the small mom-and-pop businesses had enough problems with their survival in struggling through the pandemic without the government burdening them with higher labor costs. The union leadership needs to support the candidates that support the greatest chance for economic growth. It is to grow through all our large corporations and particularly manufacturing industries.

On the night of the 2016 presidential election I was listening to a TV reporter interview an automobile worker from Michigan. The reporter asked him, "Who are you voting for?" and he said, "I and the rest of the workers on the floor are voting for Donald Trump." He said, "The boys in the union office are most likely not doing that though." Why the disconnect? Especially now, since it's clear that the radical left Socialists are making the most of our nation's policy decisions. Understand that union laborers in most cases work through the growth of the free enterprise system, our large corporations and industries, to support the personal growth of their members. This is simple government and economics. Almost every learned businessperson knows and expects to pay their labor force. With socialism, wage increases or benefits are doled out by political bureaucrats after they get their cut first. Socialism does not need unions because the government decides when and where the money is distributed.

I had the opportunity to view the Democratic National Convention (DNC) and the Republican National Convention (RNC) in 2020. It has always been interesting to me to hear what the many politicians in the United States say about how they feel about the direction our country should take or has not taken. The largest difference between the two conventions was that the DNC had the pageantry in its programming that put the greatest Rose Bowl Parade to shame. The point is, I consider myself to be a rational person when viewing TV. When I see a lot of glitter and fireworks in presentations, I have learned that it can be a distraction to the event's purpose. Every day while watching the DNC I heard about unity, closing the divide among Americans, and working together to move our nation forward. There were great, emotional, and moving speeches by the presenters. Later they announced they were unifying with the Socialist

Party. That decision by the DNC was a huge political paradigm shift to the far left. The party's control of two of the three branches of our government moved our nation to the far left. The missing branch was the Judicial Branch. I believe that is why, when Donald Trump won the presidential election in 2016, the Democratic leadership became unglued and started to call for his impeachment even before he took office. They were infuriated that during his presidency, at least two and as many as four constitutionalist Supreme Court justices might have been appointed by the incoming president, him. After the 2018 midterm change in the House of Representatives, the Democrats held a majority. It caused further frustration, because it could take years to gain total control of all three branches of our government. That would have been a Socialist's dream come true. With that control, the present two-party system in our government would have most probably been history.

For many years, the Socialists were considered to be a dangling participle or separate from the Democratic Party. However, they now have a bigger voice in party politics. The Democratic Party agreed to a political paradigm shift to the far left. In simple terms, the party's leadership took a far-left turn from their previous model, which was to be "the voice of the middle class." Why did they do this? They did it because the data from the 2016 presidential election showed that the American middle class supported the Republican candidate. In 2020, the Democratic Party began a campaign to pursue the larger industries, like Big Tech's big money, the entertainment industry, and various media, and began a more aggressive approach to further pander to black voters while adopting a hidden Socialist ideology. The huge paradigm shift to the far left eventually occurred because of the party's push to control the workings of our nation's strength, its money.

In the many months after the DNC's new unity plan I did not see a new Democratic Party working more to unify our Congress. There was not any substantial moving forward. I only witnessed a further widening and division among all Americans. Beginning in 2021, there were decisions being made by members of Congress and the administration that were not "democratic" principles at all, but were autocratic and harmful to the American middle class. The many examples were mask mandates and vaccinations for our government workers, the military, many private sector workers, and all healthcare facilities. The worst mandatory rule was keeping our children masked while in school. These mandates were still being imposed after 75 percent of all Americans had been vaccinated and COVID-19 cases continued to drop. Even when it was scientifically proven that warm weather and sunshine prevented the spread of COVID-19, the government acted to push for working at home, virtual training for our children, and more COVID testing. I understand that many people were still afraid to get COVID, but there wasn't any logical reasoning for the mandatory regulations that came down. These edicts were more likened to Socialist "undemocratic" practices rather than sound democratic ones.

The biggest problem I had with the new "regressive un-Democratic Party" was when it decided to close the Keystone pipeline and related energy sources and industries. Decreasing our energy availability while trying to crawl out of a pandemic, which caused the greatest unemployment since the 1930s Great Depression, made no good sense at all. I lived through an energy crisis in the 1970s, where we all were held hostage by OPEC (Organization of Petroleum Exporting Countries). Anyone who lived through that nightmare should have known that closing much of our energy production would lead to a constant inflationary cycle just as it had in the 1970s. Make no mistake, the shutting down of the Keystone pipeline and other energy policies *directly* caused the runaway inflation of this early decade. People were out of work, and their businesses needed all the breaks to get them back on their feet without having to face runaway inflation. It is not just about gasoline prices. It's that it takes energy to produce almost everything (supplies and transporting them), so it becomes a vicious cycle of inflation. The results from those inflationary actions caused American wage earners to lose on average, 3 percent per month of buying power in the marketplace. It is equivalent to receiving a pay cut rather than a pay increase. It was absolutely not the right time to play with energy pricing, due to cutting our ability to produce and supply products at reasonable prices. It stabbed the American middle class right in the back. It stabbed our manufacturing industries in the back too. Additionally, we will continue to pay inflated prices for commodities with respect to our incomes, regardless of whether gasoline prices drop to near 2019 prices, because marketplaces will not return to lower prices. They have already paid the labor costs to raise prices out of necessity, and there isn't any crystal ball guaranteeing any supply increases that would warrant lower prices. The inflation damage to our market prices is done no matter how gasoline prices go down in 2024. Basically, shutting down the Keystone pipeline and other energy sources has caused a cycle of inflation, individual income drain, growth loss for the middle class, and irreparable damage to our American economy.

My wife often tells me what she would tell her class of preschool children when their behavior was continuously poor. When the children would try to get her attention, she would put up a hand up and say, "Your actions are speaking so loudly that I can't hear you." How profound. It is a polite way of saying, do not bother trying to talk your way out of your rotten actions—they speak for themselves.

What we have witnessed these past few years from the Senate and the administration in their control since 2021 is bad behavior. Not just bad but unbelievably costly. The members in control would all too often make statements about losing our democracy. If you become autocratic by your actions and do not listen to your frazzled membership and continuously divide the masses with non-fiduciary actions you have become a "regressive, un-Democratic, and Far-Left Socialist Party." The one action that Socialists have repeated and done often is the continual dividing our nation on race issues and massive spending.

I mentioned in earlier chapters when discussing our nation's federal government and the Civil War that the Northern states had a total death toll of 360,222 soldiers in that four-year period. That equates to about 250 young male soldiers *dying per day* to end slavery. I'll repeat those figures for all our high school teachers and college professors: There were 250 obviously mostly white male soldiers who *died per day* to end the slavery in the Southern states. What a great sacrifice for a humanitarian cause. This is a historic fact that wasn't meant to divide anybody or anything. There should be some way to honor the aforementioned fallen and maimed Northern Civil War soldiers during the Black History Month festivities. It would be a great unifying detail for a nation that has recently seen a blitz of negative racial narratives.

I find it laughable when the new regressive, undemocratic, socialist leadership calls Republicans Nazis, racists, and white supremacists. My grandparents that immigrated from the Russian and Austro-Hungarian Empires in the 1880s did not come to the United States to join the Nazi Party. They came to the United States because they were persecuted for their religious and political beliefs. Their situation was not much different than the many immigrants who are now trying to enter into the United States illegally. The only difference is that my grandparents entered legally and did not wear T-shirts when they went through Ellis Island stating they were forever beholden to a political party for their entrance. The politicians that make up this insanity about white supremacy and Nazis should be working to get more positive things done in their areas of responsibility instead of groping for voters, or worse, inciting riots and causing chaos. The truth is people are defined by the *deeds* they do and definitely *not* by what they say! From my observations, the Democratic Party is not what its name implies. It may be printed on their banners and the party stationery letterhead, but it definitely is not democratic anymore. The party's recent actions were not just disgraceful to the American middle class, but have put our nation in jeopardy. Their actions disgraced the word *democratic* itself because many of their actions were the reverse of the word's meaning. Their undemocratic actions and methods silenced everyone about many important events with muffled mask wearing, and those same actions will take us down to the level of another third-world socialist nation. I believe the many traditional middle-class Democrats who continue to support their party are disappointed by the fact the Democratic Party agreed to the far-left paradigm shift in their party politics. However, I believe they are mostly disappointed because they were never told it was going to happen. It was a sneaky act and typically Socialist. My wife often tells me she can handle many things, but she cannot handle sneaky, backstabbing people. She says, "Once a sneak, always a sneak."

It is obvious that the majority of Americans are not in favor of the new regressive, un-Democratic Socialist Party's recent actions. The national polling agencies show this. So what are the traditional American middle-class Democrat voters supposed to do? If you refer back to chapter 17 and view the political triangle in figure 17-B, it provides a clue as to what we can do and is labeled at the bottom of the triangle. The demographics of today's politics show that it is not a linear left or right axiom, but rather triangular because of the influence of wealth, or what is called the "hierarchy of needs."

The obvious answer is to stop the propaganda lunacy by the far-left Socialist fringe, and for the Republican Party to have a political paradigm shift as well. It would be the second political paradigm shift of a political party in four years. However, it should *never* move further to the right; this is what the radical far-left Socialists plan and are "praying for" (if they know how to pray). The Republican Party must begin to shift purposely to the left and attract the forgotten traditional Democrats who are now disillusioned. These traditional Democrats need to be emancipated from the controls of their new Socialist "overseers." The Republican Party should return to and be rightfully called the "Democratic-Republican" Party, the same party that President Thomas Jefferson founded. What remains of the old Democratic Party will be the remnants of a bunch of crazy, misdirected, leaderless ideological misfits. They can call themselves whatever they want to, but please, not *democratic*.

There are three major issues the Republican Party needs to embrace in an effort to turn into this new Democratic-Republican Party. They are to first accept certain environmental causes, specifically about water-related pollutants. They need to focus on water-system safety, waste recycling, and the amount of landfill garbage, which are major concerns for our country. I did not mention air pollution and climate change because I believe it is not the time to invest in it due to the expense of the COVID-19 pandemic. A better time would be after 2030, when a wealthy China can help pay for any needed climate-change costs. Secondly, traditional conservatives should embrace the right to unionize labor, especially within large fiscally sound American corporations and industries. This helps a large portion of Americans earn higher wages. A major point here is that the Socialist method for increasing wages is to increase the minimum wage rates for everyone. This does not create better job opportunities. It creates disproportional wage rates across employment positions which may not deserve to receive them. A union's best role is when it works out of the large corporations and industries. Trade or any other labor unions have no need or use for Socialism, because in Socialism the government bureaucrats determine all wage disbursements.

Thirdly, historically Republicans do not like regulations. I can only tell you that with the stranglehold that Big-Tech's AI, our large corporations, and China have on our economy today, only through some hard and fast regulations will we be able to get out of this defenseless economic mess we are in. Sound moves by our Congress and the administration toward fair trade instead of free trade is paramount.

This chapter was the most difficult and time consuming to write. However, I believe this chapter is the most important one in this book. I hope it turns everyone's eyes from their addictive smartphones, laptops/

tablets, and TV visuals, and encourages you to begin to help our nation by helping each other. There is a song from the 1964 Broadway hit *Funny Girl*, and the lyrics go something like this: "People who need people are the luckiest people in the world." The song was written by Bob Merrill, composed by Jule Styne, and starred and was sung by Barbra Streisand.

Probably one of the most influential Americans of the latter twentieth century was Ralph Nader. He was an attorney, a champion for consumer protection, environmentalist, and believer in governmental reform. He also ran for the presidency of the United States at least three times. People like Ralph Nader, who have had causes based on sound information and facts, have made our American adventure one for the ages. He worked tirelessly to ensure that American products and services were safe. Those products and services directly improved families, unified us through sound reason, and gave our citizenry and perhaps the world hope for a better tomorrow. He was hailed as a leader by his followers and supporters. Although an ardent vocal supporter for consumer protection, it was his deeds even more than his words that earned him his great status. I am proud to say that he has been an inspiration for me throughout my professional career and now as a writer.

For this chapter, my inspiration came from the songs "A Boy Named Sue," "In the Year 2525," and "Love Train." "A Boy Named Sue" was written by Shel Silverstein and sung by Johnny Cash. "In the Year 2525" was written by Barry Richard Lee Evans and performed by Danny Zager and Barry Richard Lee Evans. "Love Train" was written by Kenneth Gamble and Leon Huff and performed by The O'Jays.

In the song "A Boy Named Sue," a young man seeks vengeance toward his father, because of the shame as Johnny Cash sings, he "gave me that awful" girl's name. I am not sure in what century the boy was named Sue. However, I can tell you that about 30 million men who listened to that Johnny Cash song in 1969 knew exactly how that boy felt about being ridiculed by having a traditional girl's name. After meeting and fighting with his father about that awful name as a young man, he finally realizes why he was named Sue. It was out of tough love, because his father was going to leave him and his mother. In 1969, we could see the humor in the song. Today, a song like this may never be written because of the media's potential ridicule over some gender issue. The second point is that men have fought in bars after a few drinks and a few differences of opinions forever. I'm not understanding the modern point about why men cannot be more manly. The question is, if testosterone supplements are being dispensed like candy, then why are men socially being more and more like dandies? There must be some other additives in those pills, or the internet really has had an unnatural brainwashing effect.

The song "In the Year 2525" takes a futuristic look into how things may be in humankind's future. I suppose the bottom line for the song is that if we don't buckle down as nations and do the right things with our technology, we'll all blow ourselves to bits. My takeaway is that we as a country can do things to improve issues in our nation and our world if we focus on and pay attention to the problems. We must discipline ourselves to manage and prioritize information, throw out or shave off the nuisance pieces, and take the time to decipher the important ones. It is difficult to offer solutions if information is purposely being held from us though. We may have four or five major cable news network sources today. However, when compared to the thousands of local news outlets, with their own journalists to report news stories as once was popular, you begin to understand how our brains are being funneled today with less and less reporting of potentially important news. The large news networks are filtering too much news today, and it is not a good thing. As for the information conduit called the internet and its brokers, Big Tech, they are too busy washing the backs of the media outlets and a political party, and therefore the information portal has become a bad, one-sided, controlled scene.

The song "Love Train" inspires hope for a peaceful and meaningful world. It inspired me to write the first supplement to this book. We should all hope for a renewed sense of direction with real obtainable goals that will get our country and our world headed in a positive direction for a brighter future. That direction is what "Love Train" is all about. We need to all join hands, just like those pastel-colored people are doing on this book's cover, and build a better tomorrow.

As I began to prepare this chapter, I found there were too many important details to cover. It would be like another book within a book. I have observed at least an additional ten topics to discuss for this chapter and this book to be considered complete. Therefore, there are ten supplements to this chapter. Nine of them will be published separately. The first one is written within this book. It is labeled "The Luv Train." The additional nine supplements are listed at the end of that supplement.

# Supplement 1:
# The Luv Train

Since 2021 we have all heard and some have seen the insane numbers of undocumented immigrants entering the United States. The majority of them are from Central and South America and the Caribbean nations. I do not know why they chose the United States, which like other countries was in the midst of a worldwide pandemic and presently is in a high inflationary period. I have my theories on the subject, but I will keep them to myself. I believe Canada may have been a good choice for them, or maybe even Belize or Mexico, since they speak the same language. I would imagine that Belize has great job opportunities in the tourism industry. However, if we take the immigration issue at face value, as it is being told or sold to us, either these people have been persecuted in their homelands and are seeking asylum, or perhaps are pursuing better job opportunities, want free medical treatment or have been paid to come to the USA. How do we fix the problem? It is a problem because governments are businesses too and have financial growth responsibilities, and democracies are fragile. I believe I have a solution to this problem though.

The aforementioned immigration of people crossing our southern border is because they understand that the United States may provide the best opportunity for a sustainable livelihood for them and their families. This may be the alternative that their homelands were unable to provide. In chapter 17 we learned that governments are businesses too. The immigrants' homelands may not have had the economic resources or management skills to provide for even the most basic human needs of their people. Those nations' economic situations may have gotten worse since the turn of the century. Not having good safe democracies and justice systems could also have played a role in this problem. Or perhaps their lands were bought off by foreign investors, like farmlands in the USA, and these immigrants were told that a condition of the property's sale was that they must go to the United States. However, I have not found any data to substantiate that, and the present administration coincidentally has not reported on either the root causes or methods to curtail immigration.

Historically under the Monroe Doctrine (December 2, 1823), and later the Organization of American States (1933), the United States was to provide security from foreign powers for any new independent nations in the western hemisphere. However, after two hundred years, the doctrine may not have performed as it possibly should have. The United States since 1823 has had domestic and international unrest, for example, our own Civil War and all the other wars up to the war in Afghanistan (see chapter 16, "War and Pieces"). The largest problem was that there never was an aggressive effort to establish a comprehensive free or fair trade for every nation in the western hemisphere, from Alaska to Chile, including the Caribbean nations. In 1993, NAFTA (North American Free Trade Agreement between Canada, Mexico, and the USA) excluded the other thirty nations that were meant to be covered by the Monroe Doctrine. Most of those nations are very needy and underdeveloped.

Ever since my first years in college I dreamed of a Greater America, one which included all thirty-three nations. It would have been a challenging and worthwhile endeavor for the United States to pursue. So much so that I thought at some future time our currency could be merged with any of these nations' currencies after they were developed. When I say *developed*, I'm referring to the same economic fibers that made and make the United States the United States. It starts with saleable commodities from each country, beginning with their staple commodities, cash crops, potential cash cows, or industries. For example, the United States' automobile industry, or Venezuela's oil industry.

This new world enterprise's initial growth would be rooted in each nation's natural resources and human capabilities. Also, reverse engineering the world's present commodities that are manufactured and distributed must be at the forefront for this venture. Many of these are commonly purchased in the USA and throughout the world. The reverse engineering would include taking our nation's largest retail chains' product lists, especially from the all-in-one big-box stores, our largest hardware stores, and even those smallest dollar stores. All products would need to be listed, item by item. We have the technical capabilities to do this. Whichever nation has the best resources for producing or manufacturing any of the items from that list would take the lead in that product's production and have that be their cash crop. The only needed trade agreement would be the guarantee itself that the listed commodities' values would be fairy distributed among the nations. The basic trade agreement is that these nations receive the opportunity and resources to build the necessary working domains—the facilities, warehousing, and distribution centers for their products.

These new domains would include the latest production technologies and be state-of-the-art. With the exception of consumables, they would produce commodities that could be repurposed if feasible. Their production methods would use less energy, waste fewer resources and materials, include recycled materials, and be able to be recycled or repurposed. The workers' wages would be transferred to their homeland banks, which would begin the monetary cycle of savings and lending. That cycle would begin monetary growth due to investments from buy-in investors.

The question is how, what, and where this growth of prosperity begins in this giant western hemisphere. I believe it starts with "the Luv Train." This new infrastructure would replace the present method of long lines of oceanic shipments of commodities from Asia. Navigable shipments would still be made to and from Caribbean island nations, but the bulk of commodities would either be grown within or manufactured in the Greater American trading market.

Probably the most important piece of the economic puzzle comes from the railway workers that would garner railway wages. Those wages should be commensurate or maybe better than the wage rates for trade labor within each of the nations. These jobs would be solid, long-term employment and not transient. The lending and availability of commodities leads to building homes, schools, hospitals, and sanitation systems. The most important aspect is the building of individual equity and the prosperity resulting from it. This can be done; it is not too late. Like the great Winston Churchill said, "Never, never give up." I'm not naïve to the many details needed for this to occur. However, I know this: We have the tools and the talent. We do need, though, to get out of the distractions from Europe or other nations' warring issues. In chapter 17 I discussed the seven M's of management. They are manpower, material, machinery, money, methods, m-powerment (empowerment), and magic (innovation, integrity, and intangibles). The one absolute need for the success of this venture is more *energy* sources.

The three most important stakeholders in this venture would be Canada, the United States, and Mexico. As growth increases in South America, Brazil and Argentina would also be key players. Canada's major involvement would be the design and operations of the railroad, because of their great railroading history and their operational skill. Any nation that can build a railroad through the Canadian Rocky Mountains would be the best for this task. The USA would help with infrastructure support, such as building locomotives, rail cars, etc. Mexico's participation would be in logistics—providing the first staging sites and the material and labor pool. Mexico's part would be much like England's was as the site for the invasion of continental Europe during WWII at Normandy, France, to beat Nazi Germany. A four-track railway system, two for passenger service and two for commercial use, would be operated by both electrical and diesel power. Each nation's capital or largest city would be a hub for passenger service, and the coastal ports would be hubs for manufacturing and commercial use.

Where does the labor for this venture come from? It comes from all thirty-three countries in the western hemisphere if they choose to be partners in this venture. However, the first choice should be given to those who need it most: the immigrants who came to the USA to work! It is clear by the high number of immigrants that they may be looking for employment opportunities. This project should resolve it, if we consider immigrants as working visitors to our nation. However, the immigrants must still consider their natural birthplace as their homeland base. I believe this "railway gateway for prosperity" is the perfect opportunity for these beleaguered immigrants. They can work if they choose on the railroads wherever they are needed, but their homeland base shall be with their nation of birth. The immigrants' service in this operation would be a very patriotic thing for those people because they may have felt discarded by their countries. It gives them an opportunity to build thriving nations. Perhaps even our own homeless citizens may find this an opportunity and a redirection of their own feelings of hopelessness. The only mandatory requirement is that everyone submit to random drug testing, as most transportation and governmental agencies require. This is because the transportation industry jobs are "safety sensitive" positions.

Who pays for the labor? An agreed system of payment could be that each of the thirty-three countries has its own branch of the Canadian National Railway System. Those workers would mostly work at their homeland railroads and be paid by those branches of the railway system. The railway branch in turn would bill those nations for the employees' labor costs. Those nations would be granted low-interest or no-interest loans by established banking institutions to help pay for the labor. The banking growth comes from the investing stockholders, benefactors, and the railroad employees' savings accounts. These saving accounts would lead to loans for building homes, schools, hospitals, and other investment enterprises.

Where do we get the energy for such a needed venture? Much of it comes from the same sources that it has in the past. However, this project will put an emphasis on solar power, where and when feasible. Every facet of the design, down to the smallest detail, should be fashioned to consider its environmental impact, especially as it relates to our world's rainforests. As the member nations grow economically, they would need to invest in a network of environmentally friendly manufacturing techniques, repurposing and recycling of paper (wood pulp), metals, and plastics. This project may require a temporary relaxation of EPA regulations in order for the USA to supply many of the needed materials. The EPA should have agents available to direct enterprising nations on how to develop and implement more environmentally friendly manufacturing methods and machinery. In essence they would be educating entrepreneurs on how to manufacture using the new methods and technologies.

The Monroe Doctrine's initial intent was to keep foreign powers from establishing footholds in the western hemisphere. The word doctrine means law. The Monroe Doctrine was an established law and should have been more forcefully executed in the past and because of that inaction needs to be enforced now more than ever. It is paramount that the initial intent be upheld. All foreign investors are welcome. However, it should only be for personal stock investments and not for foreign powers to control marketplaces or any of the governments themselves. I believe by taking the USA's economy to the migrants homelands instead of their homelands neglecting their citizen's needs, is a much better and more humanitarian response to this migration problem.

## Supplements to this Book

- Supplement 2, The audiobook and soundtrack, *2020 Visions: For Families, Friends, the Hopeful and the Helpful.*

- Supplement 3, The Controlling of Our Thoughts and Actions by Technologies and Gadgetry

- Supplement 4, The Ukraine War and Mideast Crises, The Gold Wars of World Economics and Politics

- Supplement 5, IT IS JUST MATH: WOKE (War on Kindred Entities) = 1/MAG (Make America Glorious) = TAG (Take America Down)

- Supplement 6, The Great Divide by the Un-Diverse.

- Supplement 7, The Great Demand (Not Supply) Chain Crisis

- Supplement 8, Socialism: The Hard Facts About That Soft and Fuzzy Word

- Supplement 9, How It All Began: The 1971 USA and China Trade Relationship

- Supplement 10, Ginga! Ginga! Ginga! (from the movie *Tora, Tora, Tora*).

**Chapters and Their Inspirational Songs**

Prologue – Overture:
- "Help," the Beatles
- "Raindrops Keep Falling on My Head," B.J. Thomas

Preface
- "Double Vision," Foreigner

1. Observation not Discrimination
   - "Break on Through," the Doors
2. Rights and the Right Things to Do (Acts of Kindness)
   - "For What It's Worth," Buffalo Springfield
3. Your Character, Our Country, and Our Culture
   - "Something Good" (from *The Sound of Music*)
.4. Selfishness and Vanity
   - "I Want to Talk About Me," Toby Keith
   - "You're so Vain," Carlie Simon
5. Mass Media, Social Media, and Multimedia
   - "Dirty Laundry," Don Henley
   - "It's Only Make Believe," Conway Twitty
6. Distractions to Your Goals
   - "I Can See for Miles," the Who
   - "I Can See Clearly Now," Johnny Nash
7. Our Drugged Society
   - "I Want to Take You Higher," Sly and the Family Stone
   - "Kicks," Paul Revere and the Raiders
8. When Cool Is Not So Cool
   - "In the Ghetto," Elvis Presley
   - "Straight Ahead," Jimi Hendrix
9. Religion
   - "My God," Jethro Tull
   - "I Saw God Today," George Straight
10. Men
    - "Saturday Night's Alright (For Fighting)," Elton John
    - "I'm A Man," Spencer Davis Group
11. Women
    - "The Girl from Ipanema," Astrud Gilberto
    - "Stairway to Heaven," Led Zeppelin
12. Dating, Relationships, and Premarital Activities
    - "Que Sera Sera," Doris Day
13. Marriage
    - "Waiting for a Girl Like You," Foreigner
    - "Against the Wind," Bob Seger
    - "Me and Bobby McGee," Janis Joplin

14. Family and Parenting
    - "You're Having My Baby," Paul Anka
    - "Mother's Little Helper," the Rolling Stones
    - "Cat's In the Cradle," Harry Chapin
15. Love, Hate, and Divorce
    - "Respect," Aretha Franklin
    - "You've Lost That Lovin' Feelin'," the Righteous Brothers
    - "Open Arms," Journey

Intermission – A time to reflect on helping our well-being, then others, and to ready ourselves to help our nation.
- "The Night They Drove Old Dixie Down," the Band

16. War and Pieces
    - "What's Going On," Marvin Gaye
17. Government, Economics, Politics, and Our Defense
    - "Ball of Confusion," the Temptations
    - "The Pusher," Steppenwolf
    - "Backstabbers," the O'Jays
    - "Taxman," the Beatles
    - "Sixteen Tons," Tennessee Ernie Ford
18. Our Health, Diet, Our Environment, and Pollution
    - "Nature's Way," Spirit
    - "Mother Nature's Son," the Beatles
19. Education in America
    - "The Times They Are A-Changin'," Bob Dylan
    - "Another Brick in the Wall," Pink Floyd
20. American Music: Our Legacy and Destiny
    - "Rock and Roll Heaven," the Righteous Brothers
    - "American Pie," Don McLean
21. A New Age For Reasoning
    - "Boy Named Sue," Johnny Cash
    - "In the year 2525," Zager and Evans
    - "Love Train," the O'Jays

Finis songs
- Star Spangled Banner, Jimi Hendrix
- "Revolution," the Beatles

Figure 21-A

# Endnotes

**Prologue**
1  Pope John Paul II, *Crossing the Threshold of Hope* (1997) Alfred A. Knopf Inc, p.4-5
2  The New Testament, *The New American Bible* (Lk. 1.30) p.1142

**Chapter 1**
1  "scientific method." *Merriam-Webster* 1991
2  "observation." *Merriam-Webster* 1991
3  "discrimination." *Merriam-Webster* 1991
4  "bigotry." *Merriam-Webster* 1991

**Chapter 2**
1  "Functional." *Merriam-Webster* 1991
2  "Dysfunctional." *Merriam-Webster* 1991
3  William Hillcourt, "The Official Boy Scout Handbook" in The Scout Motto, (Boy Scouts of America, 1979), 42
4  William Hillcourt, "The Official Boy Scout Handbook" in The Scout Oath or Promise, (Boy Scouts of America, 1979), 27
5  William Hillcourt, "The Official Boy Scout Handbook" in The Scout Law, (Boy Scouts of America, 1979) 31
6  The Old Testament creation story, *The New American Bible* (Ex. 20.1-17.85) p. 85

**Chapter 4**
1  "Selfish." *Merriam-Webster* 1991

**Chapter 7**
1  "stimulant." *Merriam-Webster* 1991

**Chapter 8**
1  "cool." *Merriam-Webster* 1991

**Chapter 14**
1  Benjamin Spock, M.D., *Dr. Spock's Baby and Child Care* (Gallery Books) 2018 p. 533

**Chapter 15**
1  Alexander Pope, *The Complete Poetical Works of Pope*, An Essay in Criticism (Houghton Mifflin Co. Boston) p. 74

**Chapter 17**
1  "Politics." *Merriam-Webster*, 1991 p.911
2  "Politician." *Merriam-Webster* 1991, p.911

**Chapter 18**
1  "norm." *Merriam-Webster* 1991
2  "virtual." *Merriam-Webster* 1991

www.ingramcontent.com/pod-product-compliance
Lightning Source LLC
Chambersburg PA
CBHW031152270326
41931CB00006B/243